*Birth and Death: Bioethical
Decision-Making*

Biblical Perspectives on Current Issues
HOWARD CLARK KEE, General Editor

Birth and Death: Bioethical Decision-Making

PAUL D. SIMMONS

THE WESTMINSTER PRESS

PHILADELPHIA

First edition

Published by The Westminster Press®
Philadelphia, Pennsylvania

PRINTED IN THE UNITED STATES OF AMERICA

9 8 7 6 5 4 3 2 1

Library of Congress Cataloging in Publication Data

Simmons, Paul D.
  Birth and death.

  (Biblical perspectives on current issues)
  Includes index.
  1. Medical ethics—Decision making. 2. Christian
ethics—Baptist authors. 3. Life and death, Power over—
Biblical teaching. I. Title. II. Series.
R725.5.S55 1983   174′.2   82-20160
ISBN 0-664-24463-7 (pbk.)

To

BETTY KINLAW SIMMONS

for patient understanding,
insightful counsel, and
constant encouragement

CONTENTS

EDITOR'S FOREWORD

Thoughtful persons, concerned for the future of the human race, will be challenged and informed by this book on bioethics by Dr. Paul Simmons. Drawing on a wide range of historical and contemporary resources in religion and philosophy, law and ethics, the author puts in sharp perspective the issues which our generation can avoid only at peril of extinction: Is abortion legal and morally right? Should those who want to die, or who are in inescapable misery, be allowed to die voluntarily? How much should the medical profession assist in the conception and birth of children to parents who cannot have offspring by natural means? Should biologists be permitted to engineer human genes, so as to prevent physical or behavioral disorders, or to improve the quality of the race?

As his research shows in fascinating detail, the medical skills are already available to achieve these objectives, or the research is moving rapidly to gain that kind of control over the processes of human reproduction. Should these developments be encouraged? outlawed? controlled? By careful use of the biblical traditions, Dr. Simmons shows what light the Bible may shed on these issues to the faithful seeker. He also shows how some writers have misused the Bible to support their own point of view. And further, he acknowledges that in some areas, there is no direct conclusion to be drawn from the Bible, although the basic perspectives toward human existence and moral responsibility are effectively traced for the reader.

Overarching the whole of this impressive study is the author's concern for the Christian conviction that God is working out his purpose in the world, and that the divine intention for humankind—though it has been disclosed through Jesus Christ—is yet to be fully revealed. In his fresh statement of what theologians call eschatology, Dr. Simmons declares that Christians dare not back away from scientific advances that hold out the possibility of the enrichment of human life and the overcoming of potentially horrible results of genetic changes that are already taking place in the present generations. The author also faces up to the current religious issue: evolution vs. creationism; his treatment of this question moves beyond the widespread notion that the debate is between those who are scientific in outlook and those who take the Bible seriously.

This is a provocative book. It maintains an admirable balance between mastery of the technical terminology and simple directness of expression. It should lend itself ideally not only to individual reading but also to group discussion. The issues that are presented in this volume are as controversial and as personal as any that confront our society. With the possible exception of nuclear disaster, there are no social and moral problems that raise more basic questions about the future of humanity. To avoid them would be hopelessly irresponsible. To face up to them, with the stimulus and insights of this book as a guide to weighing the issues, will be demanding, stimulating, rewarding, and informative. Those who have been inquiring along the lines of these problems will gain new perspectives. Those who disagree with Dr. Simmons will experience a forceful, yet compassionate challenge. All who wrestle with these questions under the guidance of the author will be better informed, and more fully responsible as concerned Christians.

HOWARD CLARK KEE

Boston University

Chapter 1

BIOETHICS: SCIENCE AND HUMAN VALUES

Bioethics is an area in which the interests of science and religion meet. New technologies and applied knowledge create dilemmas in the zone where technique and human values converge and often conflict. A sampling of items illustrates the problem.

An internationally known heart surgeon issues a call for legalized mercy killing. Telling of his pact with his brother and fellow surgeon and reflecting upon the recent death of his ninety-eight-year-old mother after repeated strokes complicated by pneumonia, this compassionate but skilled physician believes that the time has come to extend the artful use of medicine to enable people to die less painfully.[1]

Technology poses a moral dilemma for this physician on two fronts. First, dying patients can be kept "alive" for months (or even years), and, second, technology may help people die more quickly and without prolonged struggle. At what point should technology be applied to keep a person alive? Should it ever be used to help someone die?

Infant Doe was recently born at a hospital in Bloomington, Indiana. The child was afflicted with Down's syndrome. His esophagus was not attached to the stomach, which would cause him to die of starvation. Surgery could have corrected the digestive problem and the child's death been prevented. Were doctors morally obligated to perform that surgery? Were the parents morally justified in refusing permission for the surgery? Who should decide: hospital administrators, the physician, the courts, or the parents? Is the "right to life" the same as the "right to be kept alive"?

General Electric Corporation has been given a patent on a bacterium that eats oil.[2] Designed to aid in cleaning oil spills, the organism is the product of recombinant DNA which has fueled heated debate in such university research centers as Cambridge, Massachusetts, New Haven, Connecticut, and Princeton, New Jersey. The procedure involves splicing genes—a strand of DNA is taken from one species and inserted into another. Entirely different organisms are thus "created."

The development of a gene-splicing machine and the Supreme Court decision that such new life forms may be patented[3] have caused biogenetic laboratories to proliferate. The technique may make possible major breakthroughs in agriculture and animal husbandry. It even seems to suggest the possibility of controlling genetic deformities among people and, perhaps, of treating disease.

Such hopes are often overshadowed by fears. Some argue that uncontrollable pathogens may be created that will cause widespread suffering, death, or ecological damage. Others fear it will lead to the genetic engineering of people. If scientists can manipulate human genes and combine them with nonhuman genetic material, what will prevent them from creating people that are entirely different from the current *Homo sapiens* species or its hybrids—a cross between people and animals?

Again, the question of technique runs against the question of morality. That any number of things can be done from a technical standpoint is acknowledged. Whether they should be done is the moral question. Another thing is also certain.

Powerful forces are already in motion that will increasingly confront people with such dilemmas. The future is being shaped in the laboratories of science. The moral dilemma is whether that future will bless or curse, heal or hurt, humanity and nature. The religious question is the way in which God's will may be related to such possibilities and the future of the world.

MOMENTA TOWARD THE FUTURE

There are several sources of the momentum behind scientific developments. The first is the rapid development of technology. The development of the computer was a major breakthrough in our ability to catalog and use information. The data storage, correlation, and recall capabilities of the computer both astound and facilitate the human imagination. Patterned after the human brain in some ways, the computer now complements what people can do. It has become a partner in scientific research and applied technology.

Transistor and microcomputer technology holds even further promise for developments in the world of tomorrow. The more sophisticated the engineering techniques become, the more precise and delicate the scientific procedure that is possible. As mechanical hearts, replacement organs, modified brains, or neural systems become the objects of engineering research, a world of cyborgs is not at all unthinkable—human beings who are linked to mechanical devices for some of their vital physiological functions.

Technology, of course, has a momentum of its own.[4] When it is combined with medical research, however, the result is an exponential growth. Knowledge grows geometrically, not just arithmetically. Science doubles its information every ten years, biology every five, and genetics every two years. Scientific knowledge has doubled in the past twenty-five years. Of all scientists in history 90 percent are alive today. The past generation has witnessed 95 percent of all technological developments. The quantitative changes brought about by such activities have precipitated some of the major crises now confronting humankind. Undoubtedly, the rapidity of change can only be expected to accelerate in the future.

The second major contributor to scientific advance is a concern for human well-being. This is a dynamic that can be thought of as a moral concern for persons. Generally speaking, two concerns permeate medical science: the well-being of the patient and the common good of humanity. Science attempts to overcome the circumstances that lead to human suffering. This may take the form of therapy for the patient —curing diseases, correcting deformities, eliminating poverty and its companions, starvation and mental retardation— improving the general level of health and lengthening the life span.

The "other side" of patient therapy is *social health,* or the general well-being of society. Concern for society, for instance, is involved in the geneticist's alarm about the gene pool. Herman J. Muller has warned that "if we fail to act now to eradicate genetic defects, the job of ministering to infirmities [will] come to consume all the energy that society [can] muster for it, leaving no surplus for general cultural purposes."[5] Genetics aims to preserve the human future from its own self-destructiveness. Correcting genetic problems both aids the person and protects society.

The third component of scientific advance is curiosity. Philosophically, human beings may be regarded as creatures capable of raising questions, probing for answers, and developing skills for coping with problems. This is recognized in stories ranging from Pandora's box to the biblical account of creation, where curiosity led to the tasting of the forbidden fruit. Curiosity also has a double effect—it may lead to harmful discoveries and inventions or to knowledge and technologies that are helpful and healing. Curiosity not only "killed the cat," it also led to the discovery of electricity, gravity, and Mendelian genetics.

Other factors involved in scientific developments can also be discerned. These range from avarice to ambition. The desire for profit motivates research on chemicals or pills that will have broad acceptability and usefulness in the commercial market. Ambition also causes scientists to strive for personal or professional recognition. The high costs involved in developing drugs or in discovering cures mean that more diseases such as progeria, which causes a child to age ten times the normal rate, are simply not researched. The "user market" is simply not large enough to repay the pharmaceutical company's investment.

Personal ambition for recognition on the part of a scientist might provide motivation for such research and experimentation, but few can live without financial support and thus simply cannot afford to pursue exotic or nonprofitable goals. Ambition and competition were major forces behind research into recombinant DNA. When a financial award was offered and scientific prestige was at stake, several scientists and laboratories competed fervently for the prize.

Pure altruism hardly lies behind developments in medical science, therefore. But in their own way such research and development are thought to be for the good of humankind. Even greed for profit may be redeemed for the good of persons if cures are discovered for widespread diseases. Unadulterated ambition may be redemptive if genetic cures are discovered or made possible by new advances in recombinant DNA.

These forces taken together create a tremendous momentum toward the future. Power combines the influence of each of the tools of technology with the cumulative wisdom of the scientific community. Science is now on the verge of creating a new world—whether "brave" or "grave"[6] remains to be seen. One thing is certain, however, and that is that already we are experiencing "future shock,"[7] the numbing, chilling, and confusing effect of change that is too rapid for our proper emotional adjustment. Within a single lifetime, the world has passed through the Atomic Age, the Electronic Age, and the Space Age. Now we are entering the Age of Biotics. The questions posed by such rapid developments are baffling for both scientific and religious communities. Traditional modes of thought and values are tested and frequently found wanting. But the moral task is clear. As Van R. Potter states it forcefully:

> If we are to preserve the dignity of the individual, and if the human species is to survive and prosper, we need to cultivate the world of ideas and perfect the techniques for arriving at value judgments in areas where facts alone are not enough.[8]

BIOETHICS: DISCIPLINE FOR THE FUTURE

Bioethics, the "discipline for the future," is a study of ways to integrate moral values into the decision-making processes where technical questions may seem to be the only concern. The need can be illustrated by a conversation with the engineer in charge of the guidance system on a major nuclear project. When asked how he related his moral commitments to his work on a project that could destroy civilization, he responded by saying he had never thought of it! This devoted family man, devoutly and sincerely religious and of unquestioned integrity, was obviously concerned for moral values. But these he had isolated from his work as an engineer and physicist where the problems were dealt with as "technical" in nature.

However, because of the use of a wide variety of terms in the literature dealing with bioethical issues, certain definitions and distinctions may be helpful. This will also help to clarify the uses of these terms in this book.

Ethics is the systematic study of human moral conduct, the standards of right and wrong by which it may be directed, and the goals or goods toward which it is directed. As such, it is concerned with choices, actions, attitudes, and character. It involves an examination of the nature of the person as a moral being, the source and meaning of values in human life, and the beliefs or perspectives upon which these are based.

Christian ethics involves discerning the moral demands

and dimensions of the Christian faith. It is both descriptive and normative. Emil Brunner described it as "the science of human conduct as it is determined by divine conduct."[9] In the broadest sense it is ethical reflection carried on by one who is a Christian in the light of the biblical witness.

Historically, ethics is a branch of philosophy which seeks the truth of moral obligation under the guidance of reason. This may involve postulating the ideal human character, an effort to discover eternal ideals to which human conduct should correspond or rationally discern "the moral laws of the universe" by studying the operation of nature and history. Such studies may and will reflect schools of thought from Platonism to process philosophy.

Ethical reflection upon the particular issues raised by special areas of importance has typically been designated by the special focus of study. Thus works in political ethics, social ethics, theological ethics, or, more generally, religious ethics, etc., have appeared.

Bioethics is no exception. The term was apparently coined by Van R. Potter to refer to the moral questions being posed by the life sciences.[10] Originally applied to the ecological crisis, the term now seems to be most frequently used of the moral dilemmas posed by medicine.

Medical ethics is another term frequently associated with bioethics. It has at least three meanings: (1) a professional code of conduct, (2) moral issues in medicine, and (3) a course of study. The first refers to those principles which guide the conduct of physicians and other health care personnel. According to one definition, medical ethics is "a system of principles governing medical conduct. It deals with the relationship of a physician to the patient, the patient's family, his fellow physicians, and society at large."[11] In this sense, it may be considered as a code of professional conduct much like those used by businesses endorsed by the Chamber of Commerce. Willard Gaylin tells of his own introduction to ethics in medical school. One area dealt with the question of obligation to attend injured persons whom the physician might

happen upon in the course of playing golf. The other dealt
with promotion or publicly displaying degrees or specialties
whether in the office window or in the Yellow Pages of the
telephone directory.[12] Advertising fees or services, confiden-
tiality of patient records, questions pertaining to intimate
relations of physician and patient, and dealing with incompetent or abusive physicians have been topics of major concern.
Important as such details may be, limiting the scale of ethical
inquiry to such topics tends to trivialize the moral dimensions of medicine.

Paul Ramsey uses the term in a second and more comprehensive way to refer to the moral decisions that physicians
and/or scientists face in dealing with patients.[13] Building
upon the notion of covenant, Ramsey deals with the morality
of caring for the dying, organ transplants, and the allocation
of scarce resources.

The teaching of medical ethics has moved from what could
more accurately be called etiquette to what might legiti-
mately be called ethics. The new dilemmas of medicine and
an elevated awareness of their moral dimensions have
brought about a new era in the education of physicians. Thus,
a third use of the term is for courses that are now included
in medical school curricula designed to sensitize physicians
to the moral issues in health care and expose them to various
approaches in ethics. The purpose is to aid them in deliberat-
ing reflectively upon dilemmas now commonly confronted
so as to discern the right or proper course of action and
respond accordingly.

Behind such development lies the recognition that physicians are not simply skilled technicians charged with the
responsibility of making decisions that are technical in nature. Increasingly, it is recognized that medicine is more an
art than a science. It is also "a moral enterprise," for it deals
with the rights of persons and is involved in the enterprise
of preserving or pursuing human health and well-being.[14]

Bioethics is a much more comprehensive and far-reaching
term. It can be distinguished from medical ethics, though the

two terms cannot be separated. The latter is a special area of concern in the more inclusive concerns of bioethics which has been defined as "the systematic study of human conduct in the area of the life sciences and health care, insofar as this conduct is examined in the light of moral values and principles."[15] All the life sciences pose moral dilemmas that must be focused and dealt with. The human future is threatened by scientific "advances" on many fronts. Some of these impact upon our natural environment, producing an ecological crisis. Others threaten the survival of earth itself, as the dilemma of nuclear war demonstrates.

Physicists, architects, engineers, chemists, agriculturalists, and industrialists are other specialists whose applied knowledge poses moral issues. Thus, interdisciplinary courses of study are emerging in all technical schools. Scientific experts are brought together with specialists in ethics. They attempt to clarify the moral and technical issues, explore methods or strategies for action, and develop procedures for decision-making.[16] The effort is to move beyond the question of what *can* be done to the moral question "What ought to be done?"

THE BIBLE AND BIOETHICS

The purpose of this study is to deal with that question in the light of the biblical revelation. The issues to be examined are primarily medical in nature. Thus, "bioethics" is used interchangeably with "biomedical ethics" in order to indicate the particular area of inquiry. This is not a primer in medical ethics intended for use in a course for physicians in training. It is hoped that it will be helpful to them, for they confront those all-too-human issues both as individuals and as professionals. My aim is to examine those issues which are most prominent in the public debate and which cry out for examination from a biblical point of view.

Another purpose of this study is to examine the question of method in using the Bible to deal with issues in bioethics. This is explored in Chapter 2. The meaning of biblical authority is examined, various approaches to the Bible are explored, principles of interpretation are set forth, and the ways in which specific guidance is given are indicated. The questions of how the Bible is used and the kind of help it does provide are profoundly important. That many Christians use the Bible is indisputable. They hold it in deep respect and attempt to live by its perspectives and directions. However, how it is used or ought to be used is less certain.

The literature on bioethics is now rather extensive. Most of it deals with ethics from a philosophical perspective. Many other items of the literature are written from the perspective of Christian theology and ethics.

However, aside from a few references to scriptural passages, no book has attempted to deal with these issues from the perspective of the biblical teaching. There are small treatments on certain subjects, such as abortion, that purport to deal with the teaching of the Bible. But these do not struggle with the problem of method in biblical ethics. Further, they make no attempt to set the issue in the framework of biblical theology. Most engage in a type of proof-texting approach that operates on the basis of unexamined assumptions and frequently fails to struggle with the context and meaning of passages being cited. The end result is confusion and misdirection for Christians interested in "what the Bible says" on certain issues and incredulity on the part of those who wonder at the quantum leaps of logic and questionable exegesis. Little wonder that using the Bible in Christian ethics is regarded with much suspicion in certain circles.

Chapters 3 to 6 examine the issues of abortion, euthanasia or elective death, biotechnical parenting or artificially assisted pregnancy, and genetics. In each instance, three things are attempted. First, the issue is set in context in order to ascertain as nearly as possible the moral issues at stake. Secondly, the relevant biblical teachings are explored from a theological and ethical perspective. Finally, a posture or ethical perspective is presented that seems to be supported by the biblical witness.

Two basic but important assumptions undergird this study. The first is that the Bible not only is relevant but is indispensable for Christian ethical understandings. Not only is it unique as the historic and sacred writings of the Judeo-Christian tradition, but it is the only common reference for all Christian traditions. Thus, it has an unrivaled and indispensable place among Christians. Through the witness of the Bible, contemporary Christians are enabled to understand and follow the will of God. This notion of the truth and authority of the Bible will be explored more fully in Chapter 2.

A second major assumption is that there is no irreconcilable tension between the Bible and modern science. The divisive and often bitter debate in America over the relation of the Bible to science is both unfortunate and tragic: unfortunate because the debate is over untenable and false alternatives; tragic because the Christian faith is often masked as antiscience and the Bible as being a textbook on science.

To be sure, mistakes are being made on both sides. An uncritical biblicism is doing battle with an overly critical scientism. Each insists upon alternative views of the truth in ways and on grounds that are unacceptable to the other. I believe that both the Bible and science may contribute to our understanding of God and his will for our lives. The scientist can profit from the Scriptures; Christians who love the Bible can benefit from the perspectives of science.

For instance, science can teach us a great deal about God's world and the processes and dynamics involved in its workings. But it can neither prove nor disprove the reality of God. His ways are "past finding out" (Job 9:10). The truth of revelation does not lend itself to the scientific method of test-tube analysis, testing and verification.

The Bible can sensitize us to the working of God in nature and history. It is the product of God's revelation to people open to the transcendent reality in whom "we live and move and have our being" (Acts 17:28). It points to the purposes of God in nature and history and testifies to his creating, sustaining, and directing power. From Genesis to Revelation, God is its subject matter. It constantly reminds us that God's living presence can be experienced but not "discovered" as one does a shard on an archaeological dig or a virus under a microscope.

However, the Bible cannot and does not give us the working details of nature's processes. A great deal would be gained if the distinction between the testimony of Scripture and the witness of science were kept in mind. The Bible deals with the *who,* science deals with the *how* of nature. Conflict inevitably and rightly develops between religion and science when these distinctions are forgotten. "Scientific creationism" is bogus precisely because it is religion in the guise of science pretending that the Bible spells out the details of *how* God brought all of creation into being. Scientism is bogus precisely because it is science in the garb of religion asking the world to bow at the altar of secular theories of the ultimate origins and purposes of the universe. Conservative Christians are understandably disturbed when a scientist says that "genetic selection and environmental necessity, not God, made the species."[17] Unfortunately, some would read no farther, choosing rather to launch an attack not only on *this* scientist but on science in general and evolutionary theories in particular. Even more unfortunately, some will be so impressed as to believe the implied atheism. The end of scientism is human misery. In the armor of its vast prestige, science bestrides the modern world

> Like a Colossus; and we petty men
> Walk under his huge legs, and peep about
> To find ourselves dishonourable graves.
> (Shakespeare, *Julius Caesar* 1.2.134)

Both the Bible and science have their rightful place as servants of God. The witness of the Bible is never toward itself as the end or goal of worship. It continually points the reader toward God, the Creator and Redeemer of the universe. It is an avenue through which the ways and the will of God may be known and faithfully followed. Science too may serve the redemptive purposes of God. Its work can be worship when its investigation and application of knowledge are to the glory of God and the benefit of the world.

The Bible is not a book of science, but it should be taken seriously by scientists. It points to the sacred context in which science does its work. God as creator is also owner. Scientists may explore nature as the object of investigation, but never as owners. At best, they are stewards of the creation of God. Only creators can be owners; all others are to be faithful in their stewardship of what has been entrusted to their care.

Further, the Bible may enhance scientific appreciation for the role of subjectivity. Scientific inquiry does not deal with pure objectivity. Matter is not "just matter," nor are creatures "just creations," that may be manipulated, exploited, analyzed, and/or destroyed at will or whim. Nature has a subjective side, as both scientists and philosophers are coming to acknowledge. This is symbolized for scientists in the formula for atomic energy ($E=mc^2$), and is represented in philosophy by process thought which owes a great deal to Alfred North Whitehead. The Bible testifies to the workings and presence of God in nature whose truth is made known in varieties of ways. Nature itself becomes the bearer of the glory of God. As Elizabeth Barrett Browning rightly saw, "Earth's crammed with heaven, And every common bush afire with God" (*Aurora Leigh,* bk. vii). The supreme revelation of this truth is in the incarnation which overcomes the (false) antithesis between spiritual and material, soul and body, mind and matter. Divinity and humanity, the transcendent and the immanent, and the spiritual and the material are seen, not as inimical but as compatible realities. Each is the "other side" of the other.

This biblical perspective establishes a powerful moral constraint around the purposes and uses of scientific investigation and application. All of nature will be nourished and respected. No form of life or element of creation will be treated with contempt or needlessly exploited.

The healing arts are also given dignity and direction by our relating them to the redemptive activity of God. The biblical metaphor of Christ as physician not only embodies God's concern for the psychosomatic wholeness of the person but adds depth to the self-understanding of the health professions. Healing is a divine and human concern. Christ's miracles of restoring strength, health, and life enliven Christian support for medical science. Suffering and the limitations of disease are a challenge to this divine-human enterprise. Medicine is most effective when it deals with the person as a psychosomatic whole. Physical ailments are spiritual crises. Religious needs are as important to healing as is dealing with disease, as the story of the paralytic shows (Matt. 9:2).

Science also makes its contribution to our understanding of the Bible. It provides important filters for interpreting the message of the Bible and helps avoid certain errors that would distort or misrepresent the biblical perspective. Scientific findings regarding the antiquity of the earth and the humble beginnings of humankind, for instance, deliver us from the temptation to impose a slavish literalism upon the creation narrative. The patience and long-suffering of God (Ex. 34:6; Rom. 2:4) are underscored by the slow and torturous process by which humanity and nature have been fashioned through thousands of centuries. We are thus reminded that a "day" in Genesis 1 and 2 is not to be construed as a twenty-four-hour period. This is a dramatic metaphor conveying God's patient but powerful creative spirit bringing order out of chaos. Only human smallness and impatience (with God himself) cause us to insist that God's creative work be done on human timetables.

The truth of the Bible is not what is at stake, but the truth of our interpretation of the Bible. Insisting that the Bible is true is one thing, insisting that our interpretation of what is said is the only true and accurate interpretation is quite another. Science may aid us to avoid misreading the message of Scripture and thus distorting or misrepresenting God's revelation of himself. Not that science taught us the patience of God. The Bible itself serves as its own interpreter at this point. Genesis must be read in the light of the psalmist's insight that "one day is as a thousand years, and a thousand years as one day" in God's eternity (Ps. 90:4; II Peter 3:8). Time is a human concept and is meaningless to God.

The creation narratives are thus given fresh dimensions and liberated from the smallness of a misplaced literalism. The text should be interpreted literally as the type of material it is—a dramatic portrayal of the divine activity in creation. The passage is not descriptive science but religious drama. The human sense of awe and wonder at the marvels and mysteries of nature is deepened by the realization of the divine condescension to humankind. Psalm 8 captures that meaning when it focuses, not on *how* God created nor on the details of being human, but on the wonder of God's love for humanity.

The scope and grandeur of the cosmos are just beginning to be unfolded by science. People are still adjusting to the Copernican insight that earth is not the center of the universe. We are still trying to come to terms with what it means to be a speck of cosmic space dust living on an unpretentious planet in the corner of a relatively small galaxy on the edge of the universe. Truly to comprehend the significance of our insignificance is a human task aided by both science and the Bible. As science expands our awareness of the expansiveness of creation, the magnitude of the biblical affirmation that God loves and makes himself known to humankind is underscored. This comprehending and reflective self not only may know that it is a bit of thinking and responding space dust (Gen. 3:19b) but live in response to the Creator. In that is the glory and dignity of humankind and the greatness, love, and power of God. Truly, science may enable us better to realize our true self and thus better equip us to serve the purposes of God.

CONCLUSION

This book, then, attempts to bridge the world of thought from the biblical revelation to that of medical science. If, as Christians contend, our salvation is only from God, and the truth of God for his creatures is the subject of the biblical record, it is imperative that the Bible be related to science. This can be done most effectively, it seems to me, by thinking in two languages—theological and scientific. Alfred North Whitehead put it well: "When we consider what religion is for mankind, and what science is, it is no exaggeration to say that the future course of history depends upon the decision of this generation as to the relations between them."[18]

Skeptics in science have rejected biblical perspectives as if they are outmoded and archaic—the primitive ramblings of Iron Age ancestors. Bible-loving Christians have too often resisted science, however, as if it were the embodiment of evil, the antithesis of the ways of God in the world. I contend that Christians should resist the wedge that both groups attempt to drive between theological reflection in biblical categories and scientific investigation. The biblical affirmation is that God is one with his creation and that all truth is his to give. Thus both scientists and theologians work in God's world, both dealing with God's truth in different ways. God may reveal truth to whom he will and in his own good time. Thus, the scientist may be the bearer of a new insight from God—a new way of perceiving the world and the shaping forces of earthly life.

The other side of that equation is that a biblically informed theology can offer guidelines and perspectives that are vital to the scientific enterprise. Without the informing wisdom of values that are universally important to humankind, science will slip into an arrogance that supposes itself to be the source of human salvation. At best, it may be an instrument in the salvation of God; at worst, it can be an instrument of evil creating a destructive future for the world.

The bioethical task is vital, for scientific technology is precipitating the major moral issues confronting the world. Knowledge is power—to bless or to curse; it can be constructive or destructive; it can help or hurt. As knowledge increases, moral issues tend to become more complex and confusing. New issues about right and wrong, good and evil, desirable and undesirable are faced with urgency. Ambiguity attends deliberation and reflection. Old issues are posed in new ways. Should doctors always try to keep deformed infants alive? Should science seek to eliminate death or manipulate our genes? Can the biblical command to "be fruitful and multiply" (Gen. 1:28) be used as a warrant for scientifically aiding procreation among people?

Thoughtful Christians will resist a simple yes or no answer to such complex questions. But they will seek guidance from the Bible. Just how that may be done and the direction it provides are the concerns of this book.

Chapter 2

THE BIBLE
AND BIOETHICAL
DECISION-MAKING

The Bible is the Christian's primary source of guidance for dealing with the complex issues posed by the revolution in science. In these fascinating but disturbing areas of concern the Bible is an indispensable and reliable source of ethical wisdom. Whether the issue is genetic engineering, abortion, euthanasia, or biotechnical parenting, no other source rivals the Bible for providing direction, establishing perspectives, and developing norms for action for the Christian. The purpose of this chapter is to explore the meaning of biblical authority for bioethical decision-making. The various ways the Bible is regarded as authoritative and the differing uses of the Bible for moral guidance are also examined.

BIOETHICS AND BIBLICAL AUTHORITY

The way in which the Bible is authoritative for biomedical decisions is by no means obvious. Some writers and speakers in the area completely discount the biblical witness, considering it irrelevant. They turn to other sources of wisdom for guidance, such as philosophy, natural law, or the empirical sciences. Or, as is often the case, because of a dearth of ethical teaching in the context of medical research centers or other institutions such as universities or military laboratories, decisions are made on purely pragmatic grounds. Moral considerations are not raised. The only governing concerns may be technical (what can we do?) and financial (how can we pay for it?).

Relating the Bible to biomedical issues poses certain obvious problems. One is the lack of material in the Bible dealing with issues in medical science. Problems relating to technology and its impact on medical procedures have come into focus centuries after the last page of the Bible was written. Advances in medical science have raised issues related to life and death never anticipated by the biblical witness. Indeed, medicine itself has emerged as a science within the past three hundred years. Medical remedies in biblical times were limited largely to the use of balms (Jer. 8:22) and oils for healing (Isa. 1:6; Luke 10:34; James 5:14) and spices for embalming (John 19:40). The absence of information in the Bible about some very critical issues means that obviously the Bible cannot supply *the* answer to every problem. Both the historicity of the Bible and the incompleteness of its information are underscored at this level.

Others raise objections to certain practices recorded in the Bible and because of them dismiss the Bible as being inadequate to give guidance that could be called moral at all. Certainly by Christian standards it is impossible to justify some of the practices in the Bible. Killing an entire family because of one man's theft (Joshua 7), legalizing the execution of disobedient children (Deut. 21:18–21), sacrificing a daughter to celebrate a military victory (Judges 11), killing children for making fun of a prophet (II Kings 2:23–24), and annihilating the Amalekites to gain territory (I Samuel 15) are all examples of biblical stories that seem patently immoral. Some have found it impossible to accept as morally authoritative any book that seems to sanction such acts. The portrait of God as willing such acts is even more problematic and leads some to call it pagan or barbaric. For reasons like this, some Christians have rejected the Old Testament as authoritative.

As to the objection that the Bible does not deal with medical issues, it should be pointed out that that is hardly the

purpose of the Bible. It deals with human issues in the light
of the revelation of God. While the Bible is not a book of
science, it certainly has common interests with science as it
deals with human well-being, wholeness, and happiness. It
also deals with nature as the creation of God and thus brings
a transcendent perspective to bear upon the work of science
as a whole. The purposes of human existence as well as the
entire process of creation are placed in the context of the
revelation of God. Further, insofar as the Bible deals with
healing in the context of faith, worship, and prayer, it provides a perspective important to all of human activity, including medical science and its endeavors.

These objections also point to the historical nature of the
biblical witness. The Bible is the product of God's revealing
and redemptive activity in the midst of the historical circumstances of people attempting to understand and do his will.
They were inspired of God to address the issues of their day.
Inspiration does not remove the two major limitations of a
person's perception of God, however. People are always
creatures of finitude and they are sinners.[1] Thus their understandings were also shaped by some of the commonly held
assumptions of their day, whether social attitudes or prevailing ideas of divinity. The concept of the nature of God during
the period of the conquest and settlement was quite different
from that of the eighth-century prophets. Thus the level of
their moral insights was also considerably different. This
makes certain notions of morality that are found in the Old
Testament understandable but not normative for Christian
ethical thought.

Analyzing the various components of the moral perspectives in the Bible is a task of biblical ethics. This might be
done as a description of the moral perspectives of particular
books or groups of writings in the Bible[2] or as a more critical,
analytical, and evaluative study of the reasons behind some
of the moral opinions of the writers. Johannes Hempel, for
instance, treats the sociological factors in the ethics of ancient Israel and deals with the ideas of collectivism and objec-

tivism in ethics that would account for such acts as the slaying of Achan and his family.[3]

Other studies probe the underlying theological perspectives, such as the warrior God notions of the judges[4] and the eschatological expectations of New Testament writers[5]; a more comprehensive study deals with the interplay and influence of varieties of factors at work in the mind of the writer.[6] These focus the theological factors that both validate and provide content to the moral teachings[7] and the sociological and/or ecclesiological contexts for which such teachings were given.

The importance of such studies is threefold: (1) They recognize the integrity of the various writers and writings, allowing them to be true to their own insights and products of their own place in history; (2) they point to the interplay of various factors at work in the moral conclusions they reached; and (3) they underscore the differences that exist between biblical ethics and Christian ethics. None of the writers mentioned above assumed there is a one-to-one relationship between certain ethical perspectives in the Bible and Christian ethical norms. Plainly, there are certain passages in the Bible that are not normative for Christian thought.

In the area of biomedical issues, as with any contemporary problem, thought must move beyond descriptive studies to normative perspectives. This is the task of Christian ethics, which is the critical and analytical study of the nature of Christian faith for the purpose of articulating the types of attitudes, conduct, and actions that are appropriate to and consistent with a life commitment to God as revealed in Jesus Christ. This involves a study of the nature of persons as moral creatures, the process of moral decision-making, the sources of value, standards of conduct, and the goals or objectives of the Christian life.

The Bible is an indispensable part of that process. Bioethical issues form the agenda to be addressed; the Bible helps to provide the framework or perspective from which they

are addressed. That recognition focuses both the authoritative role of the Bible in Christian ethical formulations and the
need for a method or way of moving from Bible to ethical
conclusions.

The Authority of Scripture

At a purely descriptive level, it can confidently be said that
the biblical materials do in fact shape the theological and
moral perceptions of those who are familiar with its message
and content. Its authority rests not so much on claims made
about the Bible, nor on the fact that it is used in moral discourse, but on the fact that it actually influences our moral
judgments and actions. This functional or descriptive definition of authority is important as a corrective to those who talk
a great deal about the Bible as authority—even to the extent
of using terms such as "inerrant" and "infallible"—but do not
permit its teachings to guide their conduct or direct their
life-style. Verbal declarations to the contrary, this is to deny
biblical authority. The purpose of the Bible is not to gain
admirers for itself but to provide directions for living before
God.

Another error commonly made is the insistence that the
Bible is not authoritative for matters of doctrine or practice.
This denial may be made to avoid association with the biblicism of fundamentalism or because of perceived limitations
of the biblical witness. However, many of these persons were
molded in the life of the church and thus were influenced by
the teaching of Scripture. Insofar as the biblical material
served to aid their moral development, shape their character, and provide perspectives for reality, it has been and
continues to be authoritative for them. This is not an effort
to drag such writers into acknowledging biblical authority in
spite of their protests. Rather, it is an effort to clarify the
meaning of authority in terms of the effect of the biblical
teaching rather than on claims made about it.

Even so, the argument here being made is that the Bible
ought to be used in Christian ethical formulations. Ethics

cannot claim to be Christian that does not rely upon the Bible for normative guidance.

David H. Kelsey indicates that claims as to the authority of the Bible rest upon both functional and formal considerations.[8] First, the Bible has a unique place in the life of the church. This is to acknowledge the formal status of the Bible and the claim of the church regarding its authority. This canon is the product of the early church's judgment that this body of material authoritatively reveals the will of God.[9] This means at least two things: (1) the Bible is the book of the Christian community, the church; and (2) the Bible has revelatory value in making God's will known to people. The two hang together. The value of the Bible is not simply as literature or history but as a vital way God uses to reveal himself to the world. God may address the reader through the words of the Bible. As Leander Keck says, "The real authority of the Bible is its ability to bring about this encounter."[10] The words of Scripture may so illuminate reality that the reader responds in faith and love to the God of Scripture. This is its truth value—becoming the point of contact between the living Christ and the modern world. The fact that people continue to be confronted by God in Jesus Christ through the witness of the Bible confirms the church's contention that this is the only authoritative guide needed for its doctrine and practice. The formal claim about the authority of the Bible therefore rests upon the way the Bible actually serves to reveal the will of God. Apart from this work of God in the life of persons, any claim *about* the Bible is meaningless.

The functional authority of the Bible relates to its actual use by the church in its doctrinal and ethical formulations. Protestant Christians acknowledge the Bible as a source of influence upon their corporate and individual lives,[11] and insist that its authority is unrivaled. For Kelsey, this involves three claims: (1) that the Scriptures *ought* to be used in deriving theological and moral perspectives, (2) that the Scripture is normative, providing the standards by which

thoughts and actions are to be tested, and (3) that claims
based on the Bible establish the "Christianness" of our formulations.[12] The Bible is vital to the task of developing Christian perspectives on bioethical issues. This is not because it
is a book of science, for it does not offer an authoritative
witness in that area. Its province is the sphere of faith. It deals
with "saving knowledge," not scientific theory. In the midst
of scientific quandaries, Christians may render a faithful obedience through the guidance of Scripture.

That does not mean that Christians simply read from the
Bible in one hand and books on medical issues in the other.
The task is more complex and requires that we come to grips
with the normative elements of Scripture and apply these to
the issues we face. There are certain elements in such an
approach that can be considered by examining the question
of method in Christian ethics.

Method in Ethics

Method has to do with the way people go about making
decisions. It is an analysis of the factors or elements that play
a part in the way decisions are made. The content that one
gives to those elements determines the outcome of a decision.

One's method in ethics may be chaotic and inconsistent, or
it may be based on elements that are consciously taken into
consideration. But everyone holds certain assumptions that
give a kind of inner cohesion and consistency between what
is believed or thought to be true and the moral decisions that
are made. The task of ethics is to examine those assumptions
so that they can be dealt with consciously rather than operating as unexamined presuppositions.

This process is important for all persons, whether professional or nonprofessional in the areas of science or religion.
First of all, it aids our knowing why we believe so strongly
about certain issues. Many people know *what* they believe to
be right and wrong but they do not know *why*. Their moral
posture may be highly emotional, but they are unable to give

reasons for it beyond "That's just the way I feel!" Henry D. Aiken has referred to this as the expressive-evocative level of moral discourse.[13] The source of those strong feelings may lie in one's personal history rather than in rational beliefs that are held. A traumatic experience may do more to "lock in" a moral attitude than any moral rule or theological principle. Such people are often frustrated by not knowing why they have such strong feelings. Sometimes they create problems for an entire community of people because their arguments resist any discussion of the issues involved. Frequently they resort to religious language or appeals such as "This is the will of God!" which betrays dogmatism but does not permit dialogue.

Another value in examining method in ethics is that the level of moral discourse might be improved. Disagreement on moral issues frequently degenerates into counterproductive debates rather than a clarification of issues and better understanding between disputants. Little is to be gained when discussions about complex issues are carried on with more heat than light. Dealing with method will not rule out strongly held emotional beliefs, but it will facilitate discussion rather than diatribe. Knowing the elements in method will not only provide an agenda for discussion but will help all sides in divisive disputes to understand the opposing points of view.

A further value in methodological studies is that areas of agreement may be fashioned by an examination of the rules, principles, or philosophical-theological presuppositions that are at stake in a debate. One of the requirements for good faith in any conflict is that opponents are not seeking so much to "win" as they are seeking to know the truth. The task of ethics is to examine the moral rules or principles that one uses to justify behavior in order to determine (1) whether these rules or principles are valid, and if so, why, (2) whether these moral principles really apply to the case at hand, and (3) what principles or rules might be discovered or fashioned that do give solid guidance for the problem. Ethics forces the

discussion beyond the level of simply giving rules or principles to justify behavior to the level at which the rules themselves are subjected to analysis.

Ethics is therefore both descriptive and normative. At one
level, it simply describes what is taking place and how persons are actually thinking as they make decisions. At another
level, ethics must be critical and analytical. How were these
rules or principles derived and applied? What is their source?
Do they truly pertain to this issue? At still a further level,
ethics becomes normative by reaching conclusions based
upon the reasoning process it has employed. Norms or standards by which conduct is to be guided will be set forth.
These norms will be drawn both from goals that are to be
pursued and from the nature of certain acts. What ought to
be done may be stated in either goal-oriented or act-oriented
fashion. Or, more likely, both ends or goals and means or acts
will be important in deriving norms for action. The task of
ethics is not entirely theoretical but should lead to concrete
response based upon one's moral convictions. Ethics aims to
make those actions enlightened as well as emotional, but
enlightenment without action severs the nerve between
thought and life, mind and heart.

The final value of method is that it aids one's understanding and analysis of approaches to issues. Any writer's method
can be discerned whether or not the writer has consciously
or intentionally dealt with the question of method. Thus, one
can read or listen with greater discernment and decide for
or against a particular moral posture on the basis of the coherence, consistency, and persuasiveness of the components
involved in the argument. People are much less likely to be
stampeded into questionable or immoral behavior if they can
discern the elements upon which demagogues base their
highly persuasive but misguided appeals. Or, one may avoid
stumbling into an issue that requires an immediate decision
without having an adequate or satisfactory basis for reaching
decisions. Knowing how to think through a moral problem
helps avoid the frustration of being unprepared and of taking

actions that are inconsistent with one's religious understandings.

Discussions about method in ethics have brought to the surface several key elements. These may also be called variables, since the different content that one gives the various elements explains the differing conclusions that people reach on the same issue.[14] This is why people of integrity and good faith will still differ as to the proper moral stance regarding certain complex issues, from abortion to genetic engineering. The task is to understand those variables so that each factor can be analyzed against normative Christian judgments and biblical perspectives.

James Gustafson analyzed the debate between those who advocated a "contextual" (situational) approach and those who favored stress on "principles" in terms of four major variables.[15] These included (1) the place and importance of empirical data, (2) moral principles, (3) theological affirmations, and (4) the model of the person as moral decision maker. He pointed out that various writers may be included under the umbrella of contextualism even though they have very different starting points and models of central importance. Thus, Karl Barth was a contextualist because of his notion of the present activity of God in direct relation to the believer; Joseph Fletcher begins with the empirical data of a particular case and H. R. Niebuhr stresses the moral psychology of the believer. Niebuhr's model is that of the responsible person, immediately responsive to God and neighbor.

Likewise, Gustafson pointed out, the "principles" approach covers such diverse writers as Paul Ramsey, who uses principles drawn from natural law theory, and Carl F. H. Henry, who draws upon the moral rules of the Bible.

Gustafson made three points. First, various starting points will be found in different writers. The starting point, however, makes a difference in the nature and character of the ethical norms that are derived. Second, descriptive categories such as "contextualist" or "principlist" conceal as much as they reveal about writers, becoming almost meaningless because of the variety of approaches included under a single umbrella. Third, no matter where one begins, account must be taken of the importance of the other three base points.[16] All four areas must be included in a comprehensive approach to Christian ethics.

Glen Stassen argues the same point, though the variables he includes are slightly different. He sets forth four dimensions of decision-making: a style of moral reasoning, ground-of-meaning beliefs, faith loyalties, and perceptions of data.[17] Within each of these areas, there are critical variables or presuppositions that account for different types of decision-making and also for different conclusions regarding moral issues.

The style of moral reasoning, for instance, involves crucial differences of opinion as to the nature of rules and principles, which ones apply, and whether they are to be applied inflexibly as absolutes or more flexibly as relative to our time and place in history. Ground-of-meaning beliefs involve such questions as the nature and character of God (whether love, power, or some other concept is primary), the nature of revelation, and notions of Christian personhood. Faith loyalties and interests pose questions as to what one regards as the ultimate center of value for life and what relative values are held to be important. Perceptions of data or of the situation deal with one's understanding of threats, the locus and nature of authority, and an assessment of how change might be brought about.

USING THE BIBLE IN BIOETHICS

The interaction and interrelationship of these variables can be seen in discussions of bioethical issues that incorporate the biblical materials. The Bible shapes and our interpretation of the Bible is shaped by certain variables. One never simply uses the Bible to answer any moral question. Rather, the Bible is read through a number of "filters" that determine what is "heard" when the passage is read. *How* one reads the Bible determines to a large degree *what* one reads from the Bible. Thus, method in ethics is correlated with method in biblical studies. It is likely that one's style of moral reasoning will parallel one's style of biblical interpretation.

This can be illustrated by an examination of various uses of the Bible in ethical thought. Each approach argues that the Bible is authoritative and that one's formulations must be "biblical." Because assumptions and postures involved are so different, however, the conclusions drawn from and supported by the Bible are quite different.

The Prescriptive Approach

One approach uses the Bible as a source of moral rules or laws which are given for the concrete guidance of the faithful as they confront issues in bioethics. This has been characterized as a prescriptive approach,[18] the rules style,[19] or legalism. Doing the will of God consists in obeying the moral laws that are contained in the Bible. A moral rule is defined as a norm or standard of value stated in terms of obligation or duty. A moral law may be regarded as a command provided by God for the use of people in governing personal and social conduct. Law has also been used to designate the consistent functioning or pattern of the way the course of the world is designed or nature operates. Thus, one may speak of "the moral laws of the universe," meaning God's way of governing or directing nature. These laws no less than other rules or commands given by God are to be obeyed.

Such rules or laws are found in the commandments, precepts, and teachings of Scripture and would include paraenetic and casuistic teachings as well as apodictic commands. Doing what is right consists in obeying the moral laws of God. This approach regards the rules for behavior given to the people of biblical times as the rules for behavior for Christians of all generations.

The Bible is regarded as a collection of moral codes or the source of moral laws given by God for all people but specifically commanded for believers. The Ten Commandments, the Covenant Code, the Sermon on the Mount, and the ethical teachings in the writings of Paul all contain prescriptions or directions for behavior. Less attention is paid to the Holiness Code (Leviticus 17–26) and the Deuteronomic Code (Deuteronomy 12–28), these often being ignored or dismissed as referring only to ceremonial or ritualistic requirements not incumbent upon Christians.

The style of moral reasoning is one of seeking a rule to fit a particular moral dilemma. Decisions are made at what Stassen calls the rules level.[20] Even so, a considerable variety exists among rules-oriented ethicists, ranging from hard-line absolutism to a more moderate approach that admits that rules will often conflict. In its more extreme form, a rule is regarded as absolute and universal and thus permits no room for relativity or flexibility. Such persons deal with issues with a rigidity of style and mind-set that is unbending and frequently nonnegotiable, cutting through complexity of situation or ambiguity of values with a single, simple requirement based upon a certain rule or rules. A less extreme form is found among those who recognize that Christians may have to choose which rules to obey, since commands may conflict.

This approach to the Bible is based upon several assumptions which can be described and analyzed. For instance, revelation is regarded as the giving of objective truths about God. These are both doctrinal and moral. They are propositional statements about God and his will. Thus, the "will of God" is regarded as a group of identifiable moral rules or commands given to the people of God and recorded in Scripture. As John C. Murray argued, these are "objectively revealed precepts."[21]

Further, revelation is "closed"—God no longer speaks to his people in the same manner or with the same directness that he did to the writers of Scripture.[22] Thus, the Bible is God's final (last) word to us. Morally, therefore, the command of God is to be discerned from Scripture. The "words" of the Bible are the "words" of God and its commandments are his commands. These persons would argue that the biblical writers heard God speak to them and wrote it down.[23] They did not have to interpret what God was saying, nor did they speak out of their life situation.

Another variable is the doctrine of man or of personhood, which is dominated by the idea of sin. People are not to be trusted, because they are sinners. Reason has been tainted and warped from the Fall and inclines people to sin whenever God's rules are not obeyed explicitly.

The definition of faith or Christian belief becomes a matter of obeying the commands of God as revealed in Scripture. The contemporary follower is not responsible for intelligent discrimination, only for immediate obedience. On this basis Christian faithfulness is judged. According to Murray,

> The criterion of our standing in the kingdom of God and of reward in the age to come is nothing else than meticulous observance of the commandments of God in the minutial details of their prescription and the earnest inculcation of such observance on the part of others.[24]

A further characteristic of this approach is that it functions with a model of authority that is similar to that of the military or judicial hierarchy of power. God is portrayed as the Almighty Lawgiver and Jesus as a teacher who lays down the rule or gives orders for his disciples to follow. The definition of human responsibility follows: one is to obey the rule or law. The letter of the law becomes all-important both because "that is the way God said it" and precise obedience is the criterion for judgment.

The Deliberative Approach

The second approach also relies upon the biblical wisdom for moral direction but differs considerably in its assumptions regarding revelation and the nature of the Christian life. Edward L. Long, Jr., calls this the deliberative approach[25] which attempts to discover the universally valid but general principles set forth in Scripture. Henlee H. Barnette refers to this method as principlism in biblical ethics.[26]

This approach attempts to avoid the stock objection to rule morality, namely, that no code can be formulated that does not allow for some exceptions. The principlist seeks, not to discover the laws of the Bible, therefore, but those principles which lie behind the commandments. The principle is always morally binding, while the rule may not be. A principle is a moral value defined by reason and formulated in such a way as to express obligation. Such notions as "the dignity and worth of the person" and "the equality of all people before God" are moral principles widely shared and, many believe, deeply rooted in the biblical witness though they are never found in the Bible in precisely these terms.

Again, there is considerable variety among the ethicists who approach the Bible in this manner. Some reduce the basic principles of the biblical witness to a very few, while others expand the list to a considerable length. Andrew R. Osborne has stated the approach succinctly by saying that in the lives and teachings of Jesus and his disciples

> there is to be found a unique and authoritative statement and exemplification of the principles underlying conduct. Its method is to use the principles discovered from these sources as standards whereby to judge and interpret the facts which it has discovered from its observation of life and its analysis of the process of history.[27]

Albert Knudson reduced the principles involved in the teachings of Jesus to the principle of love and the principle of moral inwardness or moral perfection.[28]

Barnette used this method in moving from the Bible to concrete issues.[29] Behind specific commandments lie moral principles that encompass the entirety of life. Thus, the commandment forbidding the taking of God's name in vain expresses the principle of reverence for God in all deeds and words. And the commandment forbidding murder is based upon "the universal principle of the sacredness of human personality."[30]

This approach to the biblical witness is less strident than is the rules approach. The style of moral reasoning involved operates at a general principles level and then moves to a specific decision. It recognizes that cultural, time, and circumstantial differences separate us from the biblical writers. Revelation or inspiration always is conditioned by the believer's own perceptions and circumstances in history. God used the intelligence, personality, and vocabulary of the writers of Scripture. He did not just "give" doctrinal or moral statements in a certain fixed or rigid manner. Thus, in reading the Bible, the believer recognizes that specific commandments represent a particular statement of a general understanding. The reader's task is to use discriminating intelligence to discern the general moral principle at work in the mind of the writer.

This may actually enlarge the scope of a particular commandment. Barnette, for instance, argues that the commandment forbidding adultery should be taken to express the respect due the marriage bond. Thus, not only is sexual intercourse with a woman who is married to someone else forbidden, but so is any act that violates the marriage bond in any way.[31]

Another strength of this approach is that it is capable of developing biblical perspectives on current issues that may not be addressed specifically in the Bible. Thus, Barnette responded to the ecological crisis by building upon the biblical theology of creation and the principles of stewardship and Christian love.[32] Arthur Dyck develops a principlist approach to medical ethics by wedding biblical and philosophical categories.[33]

Running through every dimension of this approach are also assumptions regarding other crucial variables. The notion of faith is enlarged to include the intelligent application of Christian understandings to all of life. Faith is neither a matter of believing doctrines for which there are no rational bases nor a matter of rote obedience to rules or laws. Even though people are sinners, God gave them minds and the responsibility for using their intelligence to discern his will and make creative moral decisions.

The model of authority is also quite different from that of the rules approach. The principlist stresses the role of reason and of reasonableness. That is authoritative which is convincing or persuasive. With Luther, both Scripture *and reason* are important to Christian faith. Jesus is portrayed, not as a stern order giver, but as one who perfectly obeyed the Father by totally consecrating his mind and spirit to discovering and doing his will.

The model of the Christian life, therefore, is one that stresses the person as a decision maker using all the rational and spiritual powers at one's disposal. Responsibility is defined in terms of one's ability to think through a problem by differentiating and evaluating its many dimensions, and finally to cut through its complexities and ambiguities by formulating principles for action. Through that process the believer comes to a decision and acts upon what is thought to be right.

The biblical material is indispensable to that task and is a unique aid to the Christian's reasoning through a situation to discern and do the will of God. The biblical norms are always relevant in the midst of changing historical circumstances. But they can seldom be applied in a simple fashion. The Scriptures are appreciated no less than by the prescriptive interpreters but in a less rigid or doctrinaire way. Here there is an allegiance to and an unchallenged and irreducible place for the Bible, but it is not simply reverence for the Bible. The place and importance of human reason are underscored and brought under the scope of moral responsibility.

The Relational Approach

The third approach to the Bible to be considered may be called relational[34] or response style.[35] It stresses the response in faith which the believer is to make to the living presence of God. The Bible may certainly provide normative guidance through its specific moral teachings, but the basic consideration is the concrete response of the believer to the action and initiative of God in history. No amount of imitative behavior of the moral directives in Scripture is truly biblical until it is behavior elicited as personal response to the divine activity.

Basic to any "use" of the Bible, therefore, is one's conscious identification with the people of God. The Bible deals with the question and its answer, "How are we as the people of God to live?" This ties the believer of every age to the believers of biblical times. Their struggle with that question is the struggle of all ages. Knowing the story of how God has dealt with them enables us to enter and live that story in the ongoing of history.

The Bible is best seen, therefore, as the illuminator of the way or life-style appropriate to the people of God. Not only are the moral rules or principles helpful but so are the stories, aphorisms, models, parables, and paradigms found in the Bible. The mind is not so much a debating hall as it is a picture gallery. Not reason but response predominates. What God seeks is not so much the person who gives unthinking, unreflective obedience to rules nor the one who engages problems with cool, detached reflection, as the one who is open to the immediate leadership of the Spirit. The central task of the church in interpreting Scripture is not an objective understanding of the text but the discernment of God's will. The Scriptures are to be read in such a way that they might illuminate the believer's understanding of or evoke a commitment to doing the will of God.

The image of the person is that of one in relationship, responsive to the demands created as one confronts the other and hears the command of God to respond. Knowing what God wills may be immediate or intuitive as well as rational. Paul Lehmann, for instance, speaks of the "theonomous conscience," meaning that one may perceive what God wills by being sensitive to the activity of God.[36] And Fletcher speaks of doing what love requires in the situation in a manner that seems intuitional.[37] Faith is defined as faithfulness in relationship. It is not a matter of doctrinal conformity or obedience to rules but a relationship of trust, confidence, and obedience to the living Lord. To believe in God means to commit oneself to God in all of life, attempting to serve and follow his leadership. Christ is the supreme example of faith as obedience. He embodied the will of God and saw the superficiality of legalistically adhering to moral or ceremonial laws that actually hindered immediate responsiveness to the Father. As Jesus was related to the Father, so every believer should follow in faithful and responsive obedience.

The Bible itself is regarded as the product of human response to God's activity. Certainly it is not a record of revelation, for God's action and the person's response do not lend themselves to precise details. What God revealed and continues to reveal is the same, namely, himself. Revelation is not the disclosure of laws or rules nor even of rational principles but of the nature and character of the Creator and Redeemer. How the biblical writers expressed their experience of God depended upon many factors, including their personal vocabulary, degree of intelligence, and individual thought forms. Their perspectives were also shaped by their role, their historical circumstances, and the prevalent ideas of their day. This accounts for the variety in perspectives among the biblical writers.

A further characteristic of the relational approach is its emphasis on the fact that God is still active in history seeking to bring about his redemptive purposes. Revelation is not "closed," for God is not silent and withdrawn. Just as he called the covenant people in the past to faithful righteousness, he still calls for obedient response. God is living and active within history. The Bible testifies to a variety of forms and circumstances under which God's activity was discerned. Thus, contemporary history is still the scene of his work. The question, therefore, is not so much, "What did God command in the past?" as "What is God doing or commanding now?" It is not so much, "What does the Bible say?" argues Leonard Hodgson, as "What is God using the Bible to say?"[38] The Bible may serve to illuminate the believer's search for answers to such questions. But it never entirely or comprehensively gives the answer. The responsibility for creative discernment and faithful following remains that of the believer.

Authority in the Christian life is therefore related to experience. The Bible is authoritative as it serves to enhance or enable the believer's faithfulness to God. This may be as a result of rational deliberation or the immediacy of insightful action. Insofar as the biblical materials serve as an aid to faith, they are authoritative. Further, the authority of Jesus is not that of the giver of commands but the distinctiveness and uniqueness of his place in revelation. As the unique and unequaled revelation of the nature of God, Jesus is normative for all thought and action regarding the requirements of faith as obedience. That is a matter of relationship that can never be reduced to any rule or principle regardless of its time-tested validity or honored place in tradition.

CHRIST AND THE MORAL LIFE

Each of the three approaches to using the Bible in moral decision-making has differing assumptions or perspectives regarding the meaning of revelation, the nature of the Christian life, and models of authority and obedience. Each in its own way attempts to be faithful to the biblical witness and regards the Bible as authoritative for the Christian life. An awareness of their differing perspectives as to important variables in Christian ethical thought should enable a more careful analysis of and evaluation of the value that each approach can make to a comprehensive biblical approach to bioethical issues.

However, a careful evaluation of the various approaches is also necessary. Not every approach is of equal value, nor is it a matter of indifference as to which starting point is adopted. One of the purposes of dealing with method is to better enable people to reach decisions that are right, that are truly consistent with the will of God. We want our actions to have the quality of moral uprightness or to be supported by and consistent with our best insights as to what constitutes moral behavior. This may be stated as the desire to make our decisions "Christian," that is, consistent with our commitments to and understanding of the will of God as seen in Jesus Christ.[39]

Christ as Authority

Christ is the absolute norm by which Christians are to address all moral questions. The way in which Christ is understood as normative varies considerably among theologians and ethicists.[40] All agree, however, that Jesus is in some sense normative for ethics, for he is the unique embodiment of the will of God.[41] Understanding the role of Jesus in revelation is indispensable for understanding the essence of Christianity, which is the central question for rightly interpreting what the Bible says. One's answer to this question determines the way one construes Scripture and is decisive for the ways in which one uses the biblical materials in making decisions. Jesus Christ is the central norm by which all Scripture is to be interpreted and all "Christian" claims are to be evaluated. He is the focus of the believer's commitment, and he forms the framework for the believer's self-understanding and knowledge of God and of good and evil.[42] What we know of God in Christ relativizes and judges all other perspectives. This is seen, for instance, in the six antitheses of the Sermon on the Mount in which certain Old Testament perspectives are subordinated to those of Jesus. Thus, while the ethic of *lex talionis* (Ex. 21:23–25) was normative for the Covenant Code, the ethic of love and forgiveness is normative for Christians. Indeed the Gospel writers take pains to assert the authority of Jesus over that of any rival—whether the teachings of the lawgiver or that of the prophets (Mark 9:2–8).

Speaking of "Jesus" as norm for Christian thought and action involves a composite picture of many elements drawn from the New Testament. No one facet of his life or teaching can adequately encompass the meaning of this norm. One

component, however, is the portrait of his life-style or manner of relating to people. The attitude he embodied in his
encounters with persons and their moral dilemmas is as important as any specific injunction. His dealings with the
woman at the well in Sychar (John 4:7–26) and the woman
caught in adultery (John 8:1–11) are as instructive in regard
to the demands for a spirit of understanding, kindness, and
forgiveness, as they are for the requirements of responsibility
in sexual matters. Luke records that Jesus' hearers "won-
dered at the gracious words which proceeded out of his
mouth" (Luke 4:22). Conveying a sense of the grace of God
is as morally imperative as any commandment in Scripture.

Another factor is Jesus' teachings, including the parables
and stories that help provide vivid images and illustrations of
life in God's kingdom. These enrich the imagination and also
serve to elicit a moral response from persons familiar with
them. The cross and the resurrection are further features of
the theological-ethical portrait of Jesus as norm. These help
provide moral seriousness to the demands of discipleship and
establish the depth of commitment that love requires as well
as the basis for Christian hope.

Another feature is the apostolic witness of the early
church. In that memory other dimensions of the meaning of
Jesus for the Christian life are spelled out. Paul at times
claimed that he had a word "from the Lord" (I Cor. 11:23),
which seems to mean that he had heard Jesus teach on the
subject.

Christ and Our Use of the Bible

All these elements and more comprise what is meant in
speaking of Christ as norm for all Christian understandings.
Every posture and moral perspective that claims to be biblical must be evaluated by "Christ." This would aid Christians
to avoid several errors associated with the use of the Bible in
moral decision-making.

One is the problem of using the Bible to provide justification for patently immoral acts. The rationalization style[43]

involves using the Bible to give warrant to a particular decision whether or not the text actually says or intends the way
it is applied. This is more eisegesis (reading into the text) than
exegesis (reading out of the text). The person actually decides
on other grounds what will be done and then moves to the
Bible for a proof text. This may happen because one thinks
that others are expecting a "biblical" reason or because one
has a felt need always to use the Bible in making decisions.
It also occurs when a person with a rules style of decision-
making discovers that the Bible has no rule to cover an issue
that is being addressed. The resultant frustration may cause
the person to construe some other biblical passage to suit the
need. In any case, the text is manipulated to deal with feelings of guilt, prop up one's feelings of insecurity, or persuade
others of the rightness of a particular course of action.

   How the Bible is used is just as important as *that* it is used.
Quoting the Bible is no guarantee that one is being faithful
to the biblical revelation. Jesus' encounter with the Sad-
ducees illustrates the point. They argued that successive
marriages posed a problem for the afterlife. Jesus charged,
"You are wrong, because you know neither the scriptures
nor the power of God" (Matt. 22:29; Mark 12:24). The problem was not that they could not quote the Scriptures or were
not acquainted with their content. Their error consisted in
not rightly interpreting and applying what was read. They
wrongly interpreted the intention of God revealed in Scripture regarding marriage. They were bound to the words but
could not hear the "word" of God beyond the text. They
missed the mind of God and thus disobeyed his will even
though they quoted the words of the Bible.

   Even Satan quoted the Bible in tempting Jesus to adopt
certain strategies of leadership and thus be assured of a large
following (Matt. 4:5–6). Satan was scriptural but not truly
biblical. Some of the most demonic acts have been justified
by appeals to the Bible. Sinners and heretics have been condemned to death, "witches" have been killed, slavery has
been supported, women's rights have been denied, and un-

scrupulous business practices have been sanctioned.

The distinction between quoting the Bible and giving a biblical response is all-important. Jesus' answer to Satan both quoted Scripture and discerned the will and intention of God that are to characterize every act of genuine obedience. Discerning God's will through the words of the Bible involves "rightly dividing," "accurately handling," or "correctly presenting" and faithfully representing the word of truth (II Tim. 2:15). This can be done only if the words of the Bible are brought under the normative judgment of the Word of God and his truth in Jesus Christ (John 8:12; 14:6).

Christ as norm can also serve to aid our choosing between the relative merits of various approaches to the Bible. The style of moral reasoning as well as the content given the crucial variables must be consistent with the spirit and teachings of Jesus. This makes approaching moral issues from the perspective of the "moral laws" in the Bible terribly problematic. A major problem of this approach is that of specifying what constitutes the moral law or laws of the Bible. Certainly it goes beyond those specified in the Torah. To regard the teachings of Jesus as "law" in the same sense as those of the Old Testament is also problematic. Jesus and the lawgivers were not of the same mind. While he brought "a new law," it was one written on the heart and certainly cannot be reduced to the moral teachings of the Bible that may even have been prescriptive in their original intent. The biblical interpreter is confronted by a variety of uses of "law" in the Scripture. The various nuances and meanings must be held in mind. The unwritten and transcendent "law" of the will of God was always in tension with the "laws" as interpreted by and imposed upon the covenant community.

These problems are compounded when one examines the style of Jesus' teaching which continually brought him into conflict with those of a legalistic mind-set. Jesus' approach to moral issues contrasted strongly with that of the scribes and Pharisees. They stressed the letter of the law and the meticulous observance of ceremonial and religious requirements. For Jesus, it was not the law but the spirit of the God of grace that was to be conveyed through one's moral response. Still, he could base his call to repentance upon the laws recorded in the Old Testament where these reflected the requirements for righteousness in the kingdom.[44] Paul referred to this as "the life-giving law of the Spirit" (Rom. 8:2, NEB).

This approach is also difficult to reconcile with the Bible's insistence that love is the essence of the will of God. The Old Testament summary of God's law was that Israel "love the LORD thy God with all thine heart, and with all thy soul, and with all thy might" (Deut. 6:5; 10:12; 11:1, 13, 22; 19:9; 30:6). Both Jesus and the Jews agreed that love was the supreme commandment, though their applications were quite different. Many of the Jews were bound to the Torah as the moral content of love, while Jesus felt that love was both more demanding and less restrictive than the specifics of the law. Plainly, obedience to the law did not constitute obedience to God, as such.

The "law of love" therefore means something quite different from obeying the laws of Scripture. The apostle Paul could summarize the whole law in the single commandment of neighbor love (Gal. 5:14) and still be harshly critical of the legalistic mind-set that imprisons the spirit set free by grace (Eph. 2:8–10).

BIBLICAL GUIDANCE FOR BIOETHICAL ISSUES

What, then, is the type of guidance the Bible provides for bioethical decision-making? How can or does it serve to illuminate the issues we face?

Several things should be borne in mind. First, the Bible will not give a specific answer for every concrete case. A truly biblical approach will be open to varieties of response, for the problems we face will vary considerably in their particularity. The Bible forces us to deal with each person and every issue and to take into account all the details of which we are capable or which are available to us.

Second, the distinctiveness of the Christian response will not be in the *what* but in the *why*.[45] Christians go about making decisions pretty much as other people do. They are as dependent upon information and insight as anyone else. The difference is to be found in the informing models which they draw from the biblical revelation. Making a moral decision in medical cases is always a complex interreaction of several factors. Data from the situation and the artful application of skill and knowledge drawn from the world of medicine are brought together with religious beliefs and principles. The Christian looks to science for factual data and to the Bible for moral and theological guidance.

This also means that Christians will find areas of common agreement and interest with people who approach issues on the basis of secular philosophies or other world religions. Frequently, they will reach the same conclusions or postures regarding required or permitted acts. The distinctiveness of Christian actions is that their understanding of reality is shaped by the revelation of God in Christ and other paradigms from the biblical witness. They consciously intend the world *as Christians,* which means they will that God's intention and purpose be done in and for the world. They share the moral and theological wisdom distilled from generations of the life of the people of God. The contemporary Christian is armed with perceptions, principles, beliefs and loyalties that enable a faithful response and an ongoing witness to the living activity of God in the world. These areas can be briefly indicated.

Character and Christian Virtue

Making bioethical decisions involves both the character of the decision maker and a process of deliberation. The Bible is important in both dimensions. Its wisdom and perspectives help to shape the kind of people we are and should become,

the ideas that shape our views of reality, the moral principles
we accept, and our understanding of what it means to be the
people of God. The focus here is on the characteristics that
describe the person as a moral agent.

Being and doing are the two poles of biblical morality, for
essence and action are inseparable. One acts out of what one
is. Thus, who we are determines what we do. "You will know
them by their fruits," said Jesus. "Every sound tree bears
good fruit, but the bad tree bears evil fruit" (Matt. 7:16–17).
The Sermon on the Mount is a treatise on the ethics of being:
right conduct springs from a proper inner life (see Job 31;
Matthew 5–7.)

The supreme example of this is to be found in the incarnation. Jesus was the embodiment of the will of God. He was
said to perfectly bear the image of the Father (Col. 1:15) or
"the very stamp of his nature" (Heb. 1:3). His person and
work were so related as to be indistinguishable. What Jesus
did grew out of who he was. He thus fulfilled the purposes
of the law (Matt. 5:17) by becoming what God intended that
he be, a son perfectly committed in obedience and love (John
14:9ff.).

This is extended to all believers who are to embody or
incarnate God's will. The *imitatio Christi* motif does not call
for a slavish effort to duplicate the style of dress, manner of
speaking, or other external features of Jesus' life. Rather, it
points to Christ as the norm of all Christian life, the standard
by which the believer knows what it means to do the will of
God. As Milton L. Rudnick says, the supreme ethical norm in
the Scripture is not a moral code but a model of Christian
personhood.[46] To be Christlike is to follow Christ in doing the
will of God. Jesus' prayer for his disciples declared that he
was sending them into the world *even as he was sent* (John
17:18). This is not a missionary but an incarnational imperative. Paul appealed to the Corinthians to be imitators of him,
even as he was of Christ (I Cor. 11:1), and admonished those
in Philippi to have the same mind (spirit) in themselves as
they have in Christ (Phil. 2:5).

Doing the will of God, therefore, follows from being what God intends us to be. Lehmann speaks of God's "making and keeping human life human."[47] His model for "being human" is Christ, the truly human. Christian character takes its cue for growth toward maturity from the revelation of God in Christ.

The Bible provides specific and insightful guidance for the cultivation of virtue and the development of character. Jesus declared that his disciples "must be perfect, as your heavenly Father is perfect" (Matt. 5:48). The word for "perfect" means "whole" or "mature," and points to the responsibility of the believer to reflect or image the nature of God in one's own life. Traits of character, including dispositions, intentions, and purposes, are to be cultivated so that one's responses will embody the truth of God's revelation.[48] Biblical paraenesis, or ethical maxims and exhortations, provide helpful and specific guidance for Christian growth. This body of moral guidance represents the distilled wisdom of generations of the life of the people of God and may be found from Proverbs to James. The fruits of the Spirit (Gal. 5:22) are those moral virtues which identify and characterize those who are the people of God. The New Testament alone cites no fewer than twenty-six traits of character which should be cultivated by the faithful follower of Christ.

Self-identity is another important facet of character development. Who we are is related to *Whose* we are. Loyalties shape and define our interests and allegiances. Faith or belief is steadfast loyalty—a commitment that does not falter. It is self-conscious responsibility for and within relationship, a lived awareness of the presence and activity of God. Faith in God establishes the "center of value" around which priorities and all other loyalties are structured.[49]

The Old Covenant was premised on Israel's serving *this* God and no other (Ex. 20:2–3). The New Testament sharpens the meaning of faith by its understanding that the nature and character of God are definitively revealed in Christ. The God of Israel who is to be served is one of love and mercy. His character, made known concretely in Jesus Christ, is to be emulated in the life of his people. The indicative of his redemptive activity establishes the imperative for living for and before God. Christ thus becomes the focus of the believer's commitment. He is of supreme importance in shaping Christian identity, theology, and moral perspectives. Christ is to be made the lord of life.

Ethical Principles or Moral Action Guides

A second important area of biblical guidance is found in the moral rules and principles of the Bible. These aid the reflective task of the moral agent as concrete problems are confronted that require action or response. Statements of moral obligation among the people of God frequently took the form of commandment which expressed their understanding of God's will for their circumstances. These might be expressed as commands from God, as in the Decalogue (Ex. 20:1–17), or as a requirement for a specific problem, as in certain cases of conscience (I Corinthians 6–10). Many are expressed negatively, dealing with practices that are prohibited; others deal positively with actions required of the faithful. Some of them focus on conduct, while others deal with thoughts and motives.

Such direct guidance comprises a large portion of biblical writings. This indicates the seriousness with which God regards human conduct. His people struggled continually to discern the difference between permitted and prohibited behavior and to express that very concretely. Two things should be kept in mind. First, this does not mean that the Bible is a book of hard-and-fast rules for conduct that can be directly applied to current issues. Second, the task of moral discernment is always required of believers. Applying rules in the Bible in some mindless, unthinking fashion may do more harm than good. There are solid moral reasons why some of the rules of the Bible are not obeyed by contemporary Christians. Some are either irrelevant (such as the ceremonial laws) or raise moral issues themselves. Judging which are incumbent upon us and which are not is a necessary act of responsible faith. Part of that task involves analyzing the way the biblical writers responded in faith to their specific circumstances. Knowing the *context* of their declarations leads to a better understanding of the moral judgments they reached.

Active obedience also requires that the believer be open to the immediate work of the Spirit of God. Woodenly obeying a command in the Bible may short-circuit the leadership of God. Brunner rightly pointed to the difference in obeying the "commandments" and obeying the "command" that God may give directly.[50] Faith requires living in relationship to God, not simply living by the dictates of an ancient era in the history of the people of God.

Even so, the specific moral directives of the Bible are foundational for Christian ethics. The believer is given direction for thought and guidance for action as he or she works out the meaning and requirements of salvation (Phil. 2:12). The love commandment is the summary of God's will for human life in community. It embraces and includes all other requirements. Other rules and principles may help to explicate its meaning and apply it more specifically, but they cannot and do not rival its impact. Obeying any injunction must itself be the obedience of love. This imperative is universally valid and absolutely binding. Without love, all else is wrong (I Corinthians 13). Obeying the command to love is a matter of protecting the other, patterning one's life after God's loving acts, and intending or directing one's will toward doing the will of God.[51]

Justice is love at work seeking the effects of righteousness in community. Equity, fairness, and equal regard are all characteristics that love seeks in social policy. Justice is love serving the neighbor by using power in the political process. Excessive or destructive power is monitored and constrained for the sake of the well-being of persons. Biblical models for justice are drawn from several sources. The lawgivers sought to translate the righteousness of God into civil law; the prophets called for justice as regard for neighbor and criticized those laws which only served the interest of the powerful. In Jesus' life, the social demands of love and justice led to a confrontation with powerful business, religious, and political interests.

The biblical concern for justice guards against defining love in sentimental, emotional, or affectional terms. Primarily love is an act of the will to seek the good of the other. It is a disposition or intention to apply the standard of God's righteousness to all social relationships.

The context and requirements of love and justice were spelled out in a variety of ways by the biblical writers. The Bible is not a book of rules or a comprehensive set of solutions for cases of conscience. But it is a rich repository of moral wisdom composed of practical advice. There are specific prohibitions stated as commandments or lists of vices to avoid (Prov. 6:16ff.; Gal. 5:19–21), and positive admonitions toward behavior appropriate to and consistent with a faith commitment to God.

These commands do not give specific answers or definite formulas for every biomedical issue, of course. What love and justice require regarding abortion, euthanasia, or genetic engineering is not at all clearly spelled out. The Bible provides indispensable guidance but refuses to give detailed answers. This is both because of the distance of the biblical eras from our own and the nature of faith. We are required to accept the difficult and challenging task of discerning the will of God for our time under conditions set by complex problems in medicine and science.

Moral action guides will need to be fashioned by minds informed by the biblical witness and committed in faith to the living God. As a moral agent in the service of God, the believer translates the specific and universal commands into principles or rules of permitted or prohibited actions. That deliberative and reflective process is a unique function of personhood, bringing together rational capacities and moral commitments.

Theological Perspectives

The Bible also provides normative guidance in terms of theological perspectives. Submitting to the witness of Scripture molds one's being in the world by shaping the ideas and images by which one understands and relates to reality. As Ernest Becker says: "Beliefs about reality affect people's real actions: they help introduce the new into the world. Especially is this true for beliefs about man, about human nature and about what man may yet become."[52]

Even principles for moral action are derived from one's perceptions of God and the world. Thus the moral perspectives in the Bible must be interpreted in the light of the underlying theological beliefs or presuppositions of the writer. The debates on biomedical issues have suffered because they have often operated at the rules or principles level without the benefit of an examination of ground-of-meaning or theological perspectives.[53]

This has had unfortunate consequences. Conflicting moral claims can only be tested by an examination of the underlying theological issues. "Ultimately," says Gustafson, "a biblically-informed theology provides the basis for the final test of the validity of particular judgments."[54]

Debates in bioethics that refer to "playing God," for instance, pose theological questions as to the nature of God, the relationship of God to the world, and the place of human activity in God's work. While there is no single answer to any one of these issues in the Bible, definitive and thus authoritative perspectives are presented. These are pervasive and primary to the biblical witness and are underscored and validated in the revelation in Christ. The image of God as loving Father, for instance, is crucial for all Christian perspectives. The theological notion that God is love (I John 4:16) in both essence and action undergirds the moral imperatives that his people be loving.

The incarnation also serves to overcome the Cartesian split between spirit and matter that has haunted Christian ideas of God's relationship to the world. All that is exists and has

its being in God. Thus the entire world can become a vehicle
of the truth of God and revelatory of his nature and grace.
Creation is not simply a world of matter standing over
against God and pervaded by evil. Creation is of God and is
pervaded by his Spirit. Thus it is good both in its origin and
essence. It is also part of the redemptive activity of God, who
is bringing the entire cosmos to his promised end (Rom.
8:22f.). A theology of incarnation thus bridges the gap between spirit and matter, soul and body, transcendence and
immanence. Christ is God's truth about the world as he is
about God himself.

He is also God's truth about personhood. Debates about
"the human" in bioethics must be set in biblical perspectives.
The distinctiveness of human nature cannot be reduced to
biological factors or anatomical differences from other animals, however much these may be important or interesting.[55]

Nor is the uniquely human to be found simply in rational
capacities. The Bible relates distinctiveness to moral and
spiritual qualities. Man is always seen in relation to God, not
simply in relation to nature. Fashioned "in the image of
God," people are given responsibility for the earth from
which they are created. The person is a psychosomatic
whole, not an embodied mind or an imprisoned soul.

People are also sinners, and evil is a reality in the world.
No account of bioethical issues can escape the meaning and
importance of sin in the story of human relations to the world
and fellow creatures. Human choice can be for good or for
evil. However, discerning and acting upon the difference
belongs to moral responsibility. Where these choices affect or
are posed by human encounters with the evil in nature or
society, the issue of stewardship is focused. Human stewardship is a corollary of divine providence. God is creator and
sustainer of all that is; people cooperate with God by discerning his activity in nature and history and working to realize
his redemptive purposes. Stewardship is the care that only

people can provide, for they act under the sovereignty of divine love.

Eschatology is also crucial. The work of God in nature and history is purposive and directive. History has a goal, a telos, that God intends and commands people to pursue. This is important for the Christian vision of the world, of human nature, and God's relationship to the creative process. This image is set against those philosophies which construe history as an endless and meaningless cycle or as a static given which is as it has always been and always will be.

Human beings are stewards of the past and shapers of the future. The tools of technique not only reflect their unique personalities, but are to be used in the service of a redemptive future. People are hopers—leaning toward and anticipating the future. They live with "an eschatological itch" that moves against the evils of today, for they have a revelation of how God intends that it be tomorrow. In the biblical sense, they are the inheritors and the pursuers of God's promise for the future that is to be. That hope permeates every Christian consideration, and its importance in bioethics must be discerned.

The Place and Importance of Data

Christians are also data collectors, for no decision is responsibly made that is not adequately or accurately informed. Pious intention is no substitute for cultivated skill.

Nor can medical decisions be made simply on the basis of good morals and solid theology. The data are important for enabling one to discern the "facts" of the case insofar as that is possible. These, in turn, will be integrated into the images of reality and moral principles that one holds. That one may unplug a respirator may be stated in moral or theological terms. But that a machine *should* be unplugged or maintained must take account of the medical indicators in a given case.

The highly specific ways in which God worked in the his-

tory of his people show both that data are important and that
the biblical writers took their context seriously. Every situation is pregnant with the possibility of God's redemptive love
and purpose being shown. The human drama of the intensive
care unit reflects and captures the drama of God's care for his
world and its future.

All this comes together in the moral agent as decision
maker. Here, the elements of character, reflection, perspectives on reality, and informing facts are integrated, weighed,
and sorted through. A decision and concrete response result
from this process. When done in the context of trust and
commitment, this is faith in action, an obedient response to
the work of God under given circumstances.

There are three major components in Christian decision-
making. One is that vast array of moral guidance which one
inherits and bears as part of the people of God, the community of faith. Shared values and perspectives on reality permeate this wisdom distilled and preserved from centuries in
the life of the people of God. The second component is the
more or less objective data that are gathered as carefully and
critically as possible. This enables a reflective evaluation to
be made of the nature of the problem and alternative courses
of action to be considered. The third component is the moment of decision. Taken together, the decision is a response
in faith—before God, who is acting and willing his purpose
be pursued, and toward others, to whom we owe responsible
and caring love.

The decision itself becomes revelatory of the kind of people we are. That moment of action-response reveals the kind
of God in whom we believe, the moral values we hold to be
most important, and the way in which we embody the nature
and character of God. This helps us to understand the importance of integrity, the root meaning of which is to be integrated, to be whole or unified. The biblical word is truth.
Jesus could state, "I am the . . . truth" (John 14:6). His will was
integrated with that of the Father. So his disciples are to be
persons of integrity. This requires a commitment to research

and share informational data on the basis of truth and to act consistently with the truth of God revealed in Christ. Wherever and whenever the people of God are engaged in discussions of issues of importance, integrity of information will characterize their deliberation and discussion. Otherwise a false witness is borne that violates the revealed will of God (Ex. 20:16; Matt. 5:37). This brings together both a moral principle (regard for truth or truth-telling) and the importance of character.

CONCLUSION

The starting point for all Christian ethical action is in the person's relationship to Christ. One does not start with rules, principles, or doctrines but with relationship. On the basis of this commitment, the person uses intelligent reasoning to gather data and interpret circumstances in the light of biblical teachings and paradigms.

Finally, the prescriptive command is heard with power and authority. That rule may have been recorded in and read from the Bible. But it must be heard with conviction and applied through action. Thus, the appropriate rule for action is derived through a process of reasoning and reflection. It does not come first and thus short-circuit the reflective process.

In the following chapters, the major theological perspectives and moral principles at stake on selected issues will be examined in the light of the biblical witness. Insofar as the Bible is used or is claimed to be authoritative for contemporary perspectives, such an examination should at least sharpen the debate as to the actual content of the biblical revelation. There is no way to examine all the nondeliberative factors in the current debate, of course. These are important, but a study of the role of motives, emotional experience, and other prior-conditioning factors is elusive and beyond the scope of this work. What can be isolated for discussion and examination is those theological beliefs and moral principles which claim the Bible for their source and authority. Insofar as Christian writers appeal to the Bible to support their moral posture, those claims and the conclusions based upon them can be examined. Furthermore, the particular response or posture on these issues which seems supported by the biblical witness will be indicated.

Chapter 3

ABORTION: THE BIBLICAL AND HUMAN ISSUES

Few issues in American life are more divisive or volatile than the problem of abortion. For the past decade, it has probably been the dominant biomedical issue debated in public and in private. The subject has challenged the best legal, medical, and religious minds. There seems to be little prospect of resolving the issues to the satisfaction of everyone in this pluralistic society. Some political action groups are making a strict antiabortion stance a test for competence for public office.

Religious groups are deeply divided on the issue. Most major denominations are engaged in heated debate over the appropriate public posture with regard to abortion legislation. Some religious leaders are even linking a strict antiabortion stance with the notion of biblical inerrancy as tests for orthodoxy and Christian fellowship.[1]

The purpose of this chapter is to examine the abortion debate in the light of the biblical witness. A careful study of the biblical materials should provide positive guidance in the midst of competing claims and confusing arguments. The first need is to understand the problem in its social and historical contexts. The relevant biblical teachings on the major theological and moral issues will then be examined.

THE CONTEXT OF THE DEBATE

Abortion is a tragic theme in the story of the human race. There is pathos present in every dimension when the issue is confronted. But the human tragedy is compounded when it is played out on the political scene or when people debate it as an abstract problem with no sense of identity with the problem. The following cases help to illustrate the complexity and tragedy involved.

A forty-year-old woman has decided with her husband to have another child. They already have a five-year-old. After she is pregnant, amniocentesis is carried out because of the higher risk of fetal deformity to women her age. The fetus is deformed—badly so, the doctor said. The pregnancy is terminated. The next pregnancy resulted in a normal child.

A ten-year-old girl begins to show the signs of pregnancy. A thoughtful and concerned social worker discovered that the girl was pregnant by her grandfather who lived with the family. After talking about and weighing various alternatives, the girl requested abortion. Her parents agreed and the social worker made the arrangements. After the abortion, the girl returned to her childhood routines, her life uncomplicated by a life-threatening pregnancy and her future unhindered by the prospect of premature parenthood.

These stories could be multiplied by the dozens. Some involve fetal deformity or incest, as those above. Others involve pregnancy by rape or pregnancy of women after their children are grown and gone from home. Some involve women who are not married. Through ignorance or contraceptive failure a woman and her child now face social ostracism and traumatic adjustment in work and home relationships. The variety of reasons is kaleidoscopic. The moral and religious questions are posed for each of these in a different way, however.

The question each case addresses is whether or not it is right to terminate a pregnancy. What help might one gain from the Bible to deal with the problem of abortion? After we have set the present debate in historical perspective, several issues that are central to the debate will be examined in the light of the biblical witness.

Historical Perspectives

Historical studies indicate that women and doctors have practiced abortion virtually since the beginning of recorded history.[2] The laws of various societies ranged from the permissive to the restrictive. In either case, however, it is obvious that abortion was a reality.

Chinese documents dated approximately 2700 B.C. describe drugs that were used to induce abortion, apparently in a permissive environment. More restrictive codes were found among Semitic people. The Sumerian code of 2000 B.C., the Assyrian code of 1500 B.C., the Hammurabic and Hittite codes of 1300 B.C., and the Persian code of 600 B.C. all prohibit abortion. These codes reflect as much the attitudes toward women in the culture as the value attributed to fetal life. The Assyrian code illustrates this: "Any woman who causes to fall what her womb holds . . . shall be tried, convicted and impaled upon a stake and shall not be buried." It is interesting to note that, although the Hebrews "drew from a common background of legal jurisprudence shared throughout much of the ancient Near East,"[3] and specifically the Hammurabic code, there is no corresponding legislation that forbids abortion in the Old Testament.

The Greco-Roman world did not prohibit abortion. Philosophers recommended it for certain reasons, and physicians openly discussed potions for abortion. Plato thought abortion necessary for genetic reasons, as a means of controlling population growth and as a form of birth control for women who thought themselves too old to bear children.

Aristotle recommended abortion so that couples would not have too many children for the good of the state but said it should be done before "sensation and life," apparently a reference to "quickening" or the first movements of the fetus.[4]

Soranos of Ephesus (ca. A.D. 98–138), a famous gynecologist, discussed two types of abortifacients, *phthorion*, "which destroys what has been conceived," and *ekbolion*, "which expels what has been conceived." He went on to indicate various ways of emptying the womb or terminating pregnancy. His concern was to protect the woman, however, from any use of sharp instruments which might perforate the uterus. He also listed a number of contraceptive drugs which actually acted as abortifacients, that is, they act after the fact of conception rather than prevent conception.

The laws that restricted abortion were apparently limited to (1) abortions without the father's consent, and (2) abortions that used drugs which resulted in the death of the woman. The object of the latter was not to protect the fetus as person but to restrain those who would irresponsibly injure the woman by giving magical potions.

Abortion law reform in the Roman Empire was instigated by the early Christian church. There is no evidence of the problem emerging in biblical times. However, as Christians moved into the Mediterranean world, theological constructs were developed based on Hellenistic dualism rather than Hebrew naturalism. Christian opposition to abortion was a consequence of the developing notion of "soul" as the spiritual reality given to people to inhabit their mortal body. A corollary development was that of the evil involved in sexual intercourse, again an alien idea to the Hebrew mind. The only moral justification for coitus was that of the procreation of children. Tertullian (ca. A.D. 160–ca. 225) argued that active sexuality was pagan, while continency was Christian.[5] If procreation is the only religious justification for sexual intercourse and the soul is the divine resident in the body, abortion was a direct contradiction to the will of God.

Tertullian said that ensoulment took place as a biological

transmission from the parents to the fetus.[6] Thus, every person is linked to the original parents, Adam and Eve. This view was called "traducianism" or "generationism." Others, such as Clement of Alexandria, taught "creationism," that is, God immediately and directly creates each soul.

When the fetus became ensouled was also debated. All agreed that abortion at any time was forbidden, but it was a mortal sin to abort a fetus once it had received a rational soul. Augustine argued that "quickening" was the time of ensoulment. Aquinas, showing Aristotle's influence, said males were ensouled at forty days, females at eighty days. This became the basis for the first legislation in the Western church in 1234. The Decretals of Pope Gregory IX incorporated the notion of delayed animation or ensoulment. Laws based on the distinction between the "formed" (ensouled) and unformed fetus did not change until the impact of Mendel's genetic studies. Fertilization became the important reference point, as was seen in the 1869 pronouncement of Pope Pius IX. He declared that the direct killing of a fetus at any time was equally condemned as a mortal sin. The fetus from the time of conception is regarded as a person or human being.

In general, Luther and Calvin also opposed abortion. This was because they too largely followed natural law teachings. However, important differences in theology were developed that have contributed to an increasing divergence from traditional Roman Catholic views on abortion. Luther, for instance, refused to believe that God willed the birth or life of badly deformed infants. His struggle with the question of infant deformity was an important departure from the "nature's way" bias of natural law theory.[7] This paved the way for a very different concept of the relationship of creation and sin and thus of the way Christians may interpret God's will with regard to natural processes, such as illness or fetal deformity. Science became, for Protestants, a gift from God by which evil could better be overcome and human dominion over nature be realized.

Another revolutionary theological principle was that which stressed individual responsibility in matters of religion. Managed religion or paternalism in moral matters was contrary to the Protestant principle. A basic perspective was that the individual was directly responsible to God, not to the imperialist church or ruler. This was important to the development of religious freedom, though the Reformers did not move to that point.

The abortion reform movement in the United States during the 1960s drew upon these themes. Prior to 1969, abortion was severely restricted in all fifty states. One woman, a television personality from Arizona, had been using the tranquilizer thalidomide during early pregnancy. Reports from Europe indicated that this drug was causing severe defects in infants: hands were attached at shoulders, feet at the pelvis, and frequently facial features were severely distorted. She decided to abort but had to fly to Sweden to obtain medical help. Her life was not in danger, so no abortion was available in the United States.

Those who advocated abortion for medical reasons began to have such cases to support their cause. This was a negative effect from medical science: drugs do not always help, they sometimes create problems. The positive contribution from medicine was the technology that made abortion safe for women. The court heard evidence that restrictive abortion laws were enacted in the nineteenth century to *safeguard the health of women.* Before the advent of drugs to defeat infection and safe abortion procedures, the woman was subject to double jeopardy—the problem pregnancy and the significant risks of abortion: infection, sterilization, or death. However, with those medical breakthroughs the risk was reversed. Legal abortions in the first trimester of pregnancy became safer than childbirth. According to the *Journal of the American Medical Association* (Jan. 31, 1977), comparing deaths from pregnancy and childbirth, "legal abortion in the first trimester was nine times safer than carrying the pregnancy to term."

This referred to legal abortion services, however, not to those which were illegal. Estimates of the number of illegal abortions annually in the United States prior to 1970 ranged from 200,000 to 1,200,000. As many as 6,000 women died from abortions each year. In addition, there was widespread knowledge that the wealthy, the socially prominent, or those with influence could obtain abortions even though they were illegal. The poor relied on self-induced abortions or quack procedures that further endangered their lives. The abortion industry was called "the third largest criminal racket in the United States."[8]

Throughout history, regardless of whether abortion was disapproved by organized religion or prohibited by law, women have obtained abortions. This is not a testimony to their moral perversity nor to the wickedness of those who aided them in their plight, nor to the "paganism" of society itself, but to the human dilemma of problem pregnancy. Desperate people seek desperate and often dangerous alternatives.

These and other factors contributed to the enacting of the first reform laws which permitted abortion legally for any one of four "causes" or indications: grave risk to the life of the woman; a substantial risk to the woman's mental or physical health; radical fetal deformity; and pregnancy from rape or incest. By 1970, four states permitted abortion without requiring a showing of cause or proving the "need"—in effect, legalizing abortion on demand.

The Supreme Court Decision

On January 22, 1973, laws on abortion in this nation were significantly affected by a decision of the U.S. Supreme Court, in the case of *Roe* v. *Wade.* The Court's 7-2 decision held, in ruling on a case from Texas, that laws forbidding abortion only where the life of the mother was in danger were unconstitutional. The justices recognized: (1) the lack of consensus among religious groups regarding the fetus as person, (2) the differences among Americans regarding the proper role of laws regarding abortion, and (3) the difficulty of legislating a solution to the many complex issues surrounding requests for abortion.

Essentially, the Court adopted a compromise position that permitted states to regulate without absolutely prohibiting abortion. It held that the pregnant woman, not some other agency, was primarily responsible for the decision. The Court maintained that the Constitution does not recognize the unborn as persons in the whole sense. (Freedom of speech, vote, and the rights to "life, liberty, and the pursuit of happiness," in other words, are directed to living persons.)

The Court then attempted to strike a balance between the duty of the state to protect the woman's rights (to health care and privacy) and the conditional, more limited rights of the fetus. With regard to the woman, the Court said that her constitutional right to privacy was "broad enough to encompass [her] decision whether or not to terminate her pregnancy." However, the Court added that the state must also be concerned about the importance of potential human life. Thus, the state has the right to limit abortion when the fetus has "the moral equivalent" of personhood.

Following this reasoning, the Court ruled that abortion should be regulated according to three trimesters or stages in pregnancy. During the first trimester the woman alone, with her physician, has the full right of decision concerning abortion. The state cannot limit that choice during the first twelve weeks. In regard to the second trimester, the Court ruled that the state may pass regulations for the purpose of protecting the health of the woman who chooses to terminate her pregnancy. Thus, only competent medical personnel in approved facilities may perform abortions. However, during the last three months of pregnancy, the state can limit abortions to only those cases where the life or health of the mother is in danger. During this stage, the fetus has become "viable"—able to live on its own outside the woman's womb. Thus, the Court reasoned, in this stage the fetus is to be regarded as having the constitutional rights of persons and is to be afforded the full protection of the law.

Several things should be noted about this decision: (1) The Court did not rule that women have a constitutional right of abortion, but that they have *a right to privacy* which included decisions about a pregnancy; (2) the Court nowhere said a woman *must* have an abortion for any reasons, whether for rape, incest, fetal deformity, or any other cause —the decision is up to the woman and her physician; (3) the Court refused to establish a single solution to complex decisions during the early stages of pregnancy; (4) the Court recognized the *viable* fetus as having the constitutional status of person; (5) the question of abortion is made primarily a moral issue and not a political or legislative issue.

Thus, religious groups are left completely free to teach their parishioners whatever they wish regarding the morality of abortion and the personhood of the fetus. However, the Court refused to impose one viewpoint upon everyone, saying, in the words of Justice Harry A. Blackmun:

> We need not resolve the difficult question of when life begins. When those trained in the respective disciplines of medicine, philosophy, and theology are unable to arrive at any consensus, the judiciary at this point in the development of man's knowledge is not in a position to speculate.[9]

The Abortion Debate

Whether one supports or opposes the Supreme Court's decision depends upon attitudes one has concerning the fetus and the role of law in moral issues. A summary of the opposing points of view may be helpful. The following points will appear frequently in the argument of those who address the legal status of the question of abortion in terms of moral issues and concern. This is not intended as an exhaustive list of arguments set forth or the values at stake.[10] These are representative, however, and do recur with frequency. They are the most common issues among persons who deal with the problem on religious grounds.

Opposition to the Court's decision has been led by the Right-to-Life Movement which began as a Roman Catholic organization but now has support from persons of various religious perspectives. More recently the antiabortion movement has been given the added momentum of powerful fundamentalist religious and New Right political groups. Active at local, state, and national levels, these groups lobby for legislation to nullify the effect of the Supreme Court's decision. Their strategies include delaying tactics, legislative restrictions on availability and licensing of abortion clinics, and intimidation and/or persuasion of women contemplating abortion by blocking entrances to such facilities, lecturing the person, etc.

The final solution they seek, however, is legislative. Ultimately, a constitutional amendment is sought that would prohibit abortion for any reason except to save the life of the woman. Toward that end, members of Congress have been targeted for defeat or election on the single basis of their opposition to or support for the amendment and antiabortion goals, respectively. These groups are affluent, ambitious, and aggressive. To this point, they have made significant progress in achieving their goals. Public funding of abortions for the poor has been blocked and recent elections saw the defeat of most congressional candidates that had been targeted by these groups. This political fervor is based on religious and moral convictions which can be summarized briefly.

The basic belief is that *the conceptus is a human being in the same sense that the mother is a human being.* Thus fetus and mother are on a "par"—they are equals—in their moral value and in being persons in the fullest sense of that term. The "life" of the conceptus is regarded as the life of a human being. No distinction in the personhood of the conceptus is made at any stage from the moment of conception to the time of birth. Thus, abortion is justifiable only to save the life of the mother. That becomes a life-for-a-life situation.

A second belief is that *the willful destruction of the fetus is murder.* To destroy the embryo or fetus even in the first twelve weeks is murder, since it takes the life of a human being. Thus, the biblical commandment "You shall not kill" (Ex. 20:13) is directly applicable to abortion. Some would argue that the fetus should not be aborted even to save the life of the mother, since "better two deaths than one murder."

A third belief is that *abortion should be legally prohibited* since it is the murder of a human being. Morality should be legislated and criminal acts should be punishable by law. For them the law should protect the right to live and all property rights of the fetus.

A fourth argument focuses on what are regarded as evil consequences of relaxed laws on abortion. It is argued that *promiscuity and irresponsible sexual behavior will result from liberalized abortion laws.* Part of the concern is with the effect on nonmarried sexual practices. Others argue that couples (whether married or unmarried) may be less prudent in their use of contraceptives and rely on abortion when an unwanted, unplanned pregnancy occurs. Some argue that the Court has encouraged singles to have sexual intercourse and the girl no longer needs to fear the social and personal consequences of pregnancy outside of marriage.

Perhaps the single most important contribution of this position is the fact that it has kept alive the awareness that there is a moral issue involved in abortion. The fact that abortion has been legalized does not mean it is morally right. The question must still be posed, however, as to whether the efforts to secure a legislative solution are not misdirected. Should the *moral* decision not be made by the woman—or the couple—rather than by the courts?

Support for the Supreme Court decision comes from those persons and religious groups who believe the woman and not the state should make the primary decision about abortion. Most of the support for the Court's decision comes from persons who are affiliated with no organization. The Religious Coalition for Abortion Rights, however, is an organization that attempts to consolidate the efforts of various religious groups—Protestant, Jewish, and Roman Catholic—"to safeguard the option of legal abortion." This group does not advocate or encourage abortion but argues that a woman should have the legal right to obtain an abortion when it seems best to do so. One or more of the following arguments is usually given by those who support the Court's decision.

First, *the fetus is not to be equated with the woman as a human being.* At best, the fetus is *potentially* but not in fact a human being. Especially is this true in the earliest weeks of gestation. Distinctions as to the moral value of the conceptus are often made in terms of the stages of growth during pregnancy. The simple stages of cell division and organ differentiation hardly qualify as a person. That does not happen until the *fetus* becomes "viable," or able to live outside the womb, between the twenty-fourth and twenty-eighth week of pregnancy. At that point in development, according to this argument, the fetus may truly be regarded as a "person" or a "human being." Viability is "the moral equivalent of birth."

A second argument is that *the rights of women are denied by laws that narrowly limit the availability of abortion.* The constitutional guarantee of "equal protection" seems denied to women when more protection is given to the fetus than to the woman. Some argue that women are denied adequate medical care when they cannot obtain an abortion legally but are forced in desperate circumstances to seek help from illegal abortionists who do not use adequate health procedures. Some also maintain that restrictive laws have been passed by men who have never known the threat and terror of an unwanted pregnancy. In effect, it is argued, a woman is forced to carry a pregnancy to full term against her will.

A third argument is that *the moral issue in abortion should be separated from legislative control.* Some argue that the moral question is a matter of personal judgment—those who believe that abortion is wrong should not be required to abort for any reason; those who believe it is not wrong should not be prevented from obtaining an abortion (prior to viability). Others argue that the complexity of particular cases (deformity, rape, incest, emotional state of the woman, etc.) may be so great that an antiabortion law cannot deal with them. Or, the law becomes so complex and cumbersome that the woman is subjected to undue harassment in checking to see whether her case "qualifies." Better to leave the decision to the woman and her physician, who together can weigh the issues and decide. Apparently a vast majority of Americans support this argument.[11] According to this view, those who are trying to pass legislation against abortion are trying to impose their moral views on everyone.

A final argument is *the issue of religious freedom.* Some church-state groups have sided with the Court's decision, not because they or their constituents believe abortion is always right but because they believe in "the free exercise of religion." The definition of "person" is not a scientific matter that can be resolved by empirical data but is a theological or metaphysical question. Laws should not be based upon sectarian or religious views that are to be imposed upon everyone in a pluralistic society. The Constitution guarantees freedom *from* religious dogma as well as freedom *for* religious institutions. Narrowly defined religious dogma should not be enacted as law in the United States. Thus, antiabortion laws would be regarded as governmental "establishment of religion."

These and other arguments are used by persons who believe that abortion should be legally available. The stress is placed on the woman as the moral decision maker, and the inability of law to settle such issues for pregnant women or between religious groups who disagree on the value of the fetus prior to viability.

BIBLICAL PERSPECTIVES

The controversy over the moral acceptability of abortion will undoubtedly continue to generate heated debate in political, medical, and religious circles. At stake are opposing perspectives that lead to very different postures regarding the termination of unwanted pregnancy and the role of society in regulating these choices. The Supreme Court decision has helped to focus the basic problems to be faced in a pluralistic society. However, it has rightly refused to make normative moral judgments, leaving these to the religious community.

The Bible is used by the disputants on both sides of the abortion controversy. Each side claims that the Bible offers definitive guidance on the major questions that are to be addressed. While not all the issues that surfaced in the debate can be explored, there are certain issues that merit special attention since they are germane to the debate.

Personhood and the Fetus

Perhaps the major issue in the abortion debate centers on the question of the personhood of the fetus. Those who are working for a constitutional "human life" amendment to ban abortion in America argue that the Bible teaches (1) that the fetus is a human being, and (2) that abortion is murder and thus should be legally prohibited. According to Harold Brown:

> The Bible prohibits the taking of innocent human life. If the developing fetus is shown to be a human being . . . [or] if human life has begun, then abortion is homicide and not permissible.[12]

Though they have different starting points, many statements basically parallel the traditional Roman Catholic posture stated most forcibly by Pope Pius XII:

> Innocent human life, in whatever condition it is found, is withdrawn, from the very first moment of its existence, from any direct deliberate attack. This is a fundamental right of the human person, which is of general value in the Christian conception of life; hence as valid for the life still hidden within the womb of the mother as for the life already born and developing outside of her; as much opposed to direct abortion as to the direct killing of the child before, during or after its birth.[13]

Karl Barth is also frequently quoted:

> No pretext can alter the fact that the whole circle of those concerned is in the strict sense engaged in the killing of human life. For the unborn child is from the very first a child. It is still developing and has no independent life. But it is a man and not a thing, nor a mere part of the mother's body.[14]

Not all scholars are convinced the Bible teaches that abortion is murder or that the fetus is a person. John Stott, for instance, rejects the notion that a fetus is a human being; he believes that, at best, it may be regarded as potentially a person.[15]

Several things might be noted about these statements. First, many writers use the terms "human," "human life," "life," "person," and "human being" as if they were synonymous and thus interchangeable. Second, each statement reveals certain assumptions about what it means to be a human being or person. Third, each writer brings the teaching of the Bible as that writer understands it to buttress the argument. Finally, there is apparently no single teaching or definition in the Bible regarding personhood, or there would presumably be universal agreement among biblical scholars on this question. To understand the question of the personhood of the fetus and relate the teaching of the Bible more clearly to the question, it may prove helpful to deal with some of the assumptions involved.

Stages of Fetal Development. There is a scientific consensus regarding fetal development that is important to understand. The life of any particular person is on a continuum from the time of conception to death. There are four stages in the development of the fetus. The *zygote* is the female ovum (egg) that has been fertilized by the male sperm in the Fallopian tubes of the woman, where it remains for about three days. During this time, cell division begins. The *blastocyst* is the stage begun with implantation in the uterus, where rapid cell division continues. Many zygotes never attach, of course, and pass unnoticed through the woman's menses. The *embryo* is the stage beginning after two weeks from conception. During this time there is organ differentiation. All the internal organs one will ever have are present in rudimentary form by the end of six weeks. The *fetus* is the stage from eight weeks to birth, during which there is continuous growth or development but nothing "new" is added. This is the period of bringing to readiness for birth what is already begun.

Certainly all agree that there is a biological basis for human personality. These beginnings, however tentative or elementary, are basic to the more completely developed product, the person. This fact causes some to focus almost exclusively upon a biological definition of personhood equating "person" with some stage in this developmental process or the acquisition of some factor without which there would be no such thing as a person. Others combine elements of biological development with relational or social factors.

Three Schools of Thought. Daniel Callahan has shown that there are basically three approaches to the question of the human status of the fetus.[16]

The genetic school identifies the person with the person's genetic code. Every person's physical and mental endowments are "coded" with the combination of the female ovum and the male sperm. Genes and chromosomes decide everything from the color of hair and eyes to the glands that govern body chemistry. Since the genetic code of the conceptus is different from that of the pregnant woman, it is a person, some argue. Thus, Paul Ramsey says:

> It might be said that in all essential respects the individual is whoever he is going to become from the moment of impregnation. . . . Subsequent development cannot be described as becoming something he is not now. It can only be described as a process of achieving, a process of becoming what he already is. Genetics teaches us that we were from the beginning what we essentially still are in every cell and in every generally human attribute and in every individual attribute.[17]

The developmental school argues that genotype is not enough—there must be more physiological capacity before it is meaningful to speak of the fetus as person. Opinion divides over how much development is needed and thus at what point the fetus may be considered a person. The argument is somewhat similar to earlier distinctions between the "formed" and "unformed" fetus. Some focus on implantation. Others on organ differentiation. Still others consider quickening or movement necessary, since the "presence" and "otherness" of the fetus are then established. Many regard viability as the necessary stage, since true independence from the woman is established biologically as well as genetically. Also, the brain and other organs are sufficiently developed to speak meaningfully of capacities, not just potentialities.

The social consequences school focuses on social and relational factors in personhood or argues that society will establish the definition of person. For them, life cannot be limited to biological factors but must be considered qualitatively. Being a person involves more than vital functions, however important and basic to living these might be. Well-being, happiness, a sense of purpose and meaning, all are a part of being a human being.

As for the fetus, this group would contend that its value is extrinsic, not intrinsic. Society will decide what value to place upon fetal life, by defining what human is. Some combine the quality of life notion with the family context and personal moral value structures of the parents responsible for the fetus. Jürgen Moltmann makes a distinction between the destruction of the *vitality* and the destruction of *humanity* in the fetus. For him, the origin of humanity is not in biological beginnings but in the atmosphere of acceptance and recognition by others, since it belongs to the essence of human life that it is *accepted* and *affirmed, recognized* and *loved.*"[18] Abortion is a question of values, not of vital life signs. The nurturing atmosphere of the human family is essential to becoming a person. Thus, if the parents regard the fetus as human, it has that moral value and will be nurtured to personhood.

Generally speaking, attitudes toward abortion can be correlated with these approaches. Those who take the developmental approach are not likely to regard every abortion as the destruction of a person. They would disagree over the time during gestation at which that would be true, however. The social consequences approach would largely leave the decision to the woman or the couple involved, believing that their moral attitudes would serve as the primary protection of fetal life. Those who begin with the genetic definition, however, feel that no abortion can be morally justified, for it is the murder of a person. This approach has the value of establishing an objective standard or point of reference (conception) that can be universally recognized by morals, law, and medicine. This gives its proponents the decided advantage of simplicity in arguing their case. Each of the other approaches is much more difficult to apply to legal or medical considerations.

Simplicity of understanding and ease of application are hardly tests of its theological or moral adequacy or accuracy, however. There are logical, moral, and biblical-theological reasons for not accepting the easy equating of fetus with person.

Logically, for instance, no one can deny the continuum from fertilization to maturity and adulthood. That does not mean, however, that every step on the continuum has the same value or constitutes the same entity. A good analogy is that of a fertilized hen egg. The DNA, or genetic code, of a chicken is established with fertilization. Given the proper incubation environment, the egg will become a chicken and the chick will grow to be a hen or a rooster. However, no rational person is confused about the entity he or she is eating when eggs are served for breakfast. An egg—even a fertilized egg—is an egg and not a chicken.

Further, the genetic definition confuses potentialities with actualities. Potential entities are certainly important but they do not have the same value—moral or otherwise—as actual entities. As Charles Hartshorne argued: "An embryo is not a person but the possibility of there being a person many months or even years in the future. Obviously, possibilities are important but to blur the distinction between them and actualities is to darken counsel."[19] Thus, says Stott, the decision to abort is a choice between an actual human being (the woman) and a potential human being.[20]

Sissela Bok has said that the claim that a conceptus is a human being is based upon "a premature ultimate"—claiming an absolute value for what has only relative moral worth.[21] People have an ultimate value in Western morality but fetuses do not. Certainly the unborn fetus has moral value, but it is not of equal value with actual persons, in particular, the pregnant woman.

The logical fallacy of this definition of person is also seen when the argument is reduced *ad absurdum*. Every body cell of a person contains the person's genetic code. This is why, theoretically, at least, scientists think cloning or duplicating a person may be possible. Using the genetic definition of person, however, would mean regarding each body cell as a human being, since each cell has the potentiality for becoming another person through cloning. The implications of this line of reasoning for surgery—even the excising of cancer cells—is staggering and frightening.

The fatal weakness of this position is its radical reductionism. The easy equating of "person" with "fertilized ovum" (zygote) moves from a terribly complex entity to an irreducible minimum. A zygote is a cluster of cells but hardly complex or developed enough to be considered a person. The creature called person has capacities of reflective choice, relations with others, social experience, moral perception, and self-awareness, among others.[22] Both the person and the zygote have "life" and both are "human," since they belong to *Homo sapiens*. But a zygote or a blastocyst does not embody the qualities that pertain to personhood. A great deal more complex development and growth are necessary before the attributes of "person" are acquired.

The Bible and the Fetus. This distinction seems basic to the story in Ex. 21:22–25—an important passage for those who are interested in biblical perspectives on the abortion question. This is an account of a pregnant woman who becomes involved in a brawl between two men and has a miscarriage. A distinction is then made between the penalty that is to be exacted for the loss of the fetus and any injury to the woman. For the fetus, a fine is paid as determined by the husband and the judges (v. 22). However, if the woman is injured or dies, the law of punishment in kind *(lex talionis)* is applied: "Thou shalt give life for life, eye for eye, tooth for tooth, hand for hand, foot for foot, burning for burning, wound for wound, stripe for stripe" (vs. 23–25).

The story has only limited application to the current abortion debate, since it deals with accidental, not willful, pregnancy termination. Even so, the distinction made between the protection accorded the woman and that accorded the fetus under covenant law is important. The woman has full standing as a person under the covenant, the fetus has only a relative standing, certainly inferior to that of the woman. This passage gives no support to the parity argument that gives equal religious and moral worth to woman and fetus. The variation in the penalty levied reveals a clear distinction between the fetus in the womb and people included under covenant protection.

Jack W. Cottrell challenges this view, saying that parity is actually assumed by the passage. His argument is that v. 22 refers to the early birth of an otherwise healthy child (no harm), and that *lex talionis* applies to both fetus and mother in case of injury. "What is contrasted," he says, "is a situation in which harm comes to neither mother nor child, and a situation in which either one or the other is harmed."[23] His argument has been quite influential among evangelicals on the abortion issue.

However, his interpretation seems to force an argument

that the text itself will not support. Three things should be noted. First, by his own admission he stands virtually alone among scholarly translators and interpreters of this text. Second, the Talmud sees v. 21 as a miscarriage, equivalent to a property loss by the father. The fine levied is regarded as compensation for pain to the woman and for the value of the embryo to her husband.

Third, Cottrell concludes his study of this passage by saying that "God considers the unborn child fully human." However, one can hardly derive a theology or even a statement of personhood from this passage. The biblical writer was not dealing with such a complex question. He is treating only those regulations which pertain to the covenant community. This is not a statement about their personhood (as with slaves, oxen, etc.) but about punishment for accidents or injuries. The most that can be said from this passage is that a distinction in value is made. Both fetus and woman had value, but not equal value and thus not equal protection. Bruce K. Waltke notes that Lev. 24:17 requires the death penalty for anyone who "kills any human life," and says that this plainly is not the case in Exodus 21 for causing the death of the fetus. He concludes that the fetus is not reckoned as a soul in the Old Testament.[24]

The Biblical View of Person. The Old Testament does not begin with careful instruction about the meaning of personhood, nor does it give an explanation of conception. Rather, the biblical writers deal with images of personhood. The portrait of person begins in the creation of Adam and Eve. God created man as male and female. Three texts are of critical importance. Genesis 2:7 declares: "The LORD God formed man of the dust of the ground, and breathed into his nostrils the breath of life; and man became a living soul." The biological aspects of personhood are metaphorically portrayed in terms of "dust" or "clay." God as the origin and giver of life is captured by his breathing life into the clay he has fashioned. The declaration "became a living soul" designates the person as animated flesh. As the person is breathed into, so the person breathes. This became the basis for the development of the Jewish notion that only when a child was born and took the first breath did the child become a living soul, i.e., a person.

The second text distinguishes persons from the animal creation. Genesis 1:26–28 declares that "God created man in his own image, in the image of God he created him." The biblical portrait of person centers in the notion of the image of God. This is not a physical likeness but a similarity of powers or abilities. Francis Schaeffer and Harold Brown[25] speak of the image of God almost in terms of substance or the possession of some faculty which gives special status before God.[26]

They leave the impression that this image is similar to what the ancients spoke of as the divine spark in persons; it is an entity separable from but residing in the person. The biblical concept is quite different, for it focuses on capacities or characteristics that define the person as person and thus as bearers of the image of God. These are not infused or divine entities but are functions of what it means to be a creature who reflects godlike abilities. These capacities or powers are spiritual, personal, relational, moral, and intellectual. Of all the creatures fashioned by God, only people are able to relate to the creator in obedience or rebellion. Only they experience the godlike powers of self-transcendence and self-awareness. This creature, like God, is introspective, retrospective, and prospective. This one may reflect upon the past, anticipate the future, and discern the activity of God in his or her personal life and history.

The third text portrays the person as a moral decision maker. In Gen. 3:22, God says: "Behold, the man is become as one of us, to know good and evil." To be a person is to be a choice maker, reflecting God's own ability to distinguish good from evil, right from wrong. This does not mean that people have perfect knowledge of right and wrong as some intrinsic gift from birth. Decisions must be made on the basis of one's understanding of God's will. The fact that they ate "of the tree of the knowledge of good and evil" means that people are given the burden and responsibility of making decisions that reflect their unique place in God's creation.

To be a person is to be an agent or actor, able to exercise judgments in keeping with purposes, rules, values, and ends that are moral in nature. Imaging the powers of God himself, people are able to enter the course of history and direct a course of events. They can be relatively free from the constraints of instinct—a freedom made possible by the ability to reflect upon and evaluate circumstances and events and decide a course of action.

Thus, God is truly pro-choice. Of all his creatures, only one bears his image that makes choice-making possible. No wonder the biblical writers celebrated the creation of man and woman as the height of all creation. God's activity in creation and history is to bring life into being which can relate consciously to him and make choices in keeping with his will. God is for life but supremely for life that is able to make choices.

The biblical portrait of person, therefore, is that of a complex, many-sided creature with the godlike ability and responsibility of making choices. The fetus—certainly in the early stages of gestation—hardly meets those characteristics. At best, it begins to attain those biological basics which are necessary to show such capacities no earlier than the latter part of gestation. The "burden of proof" argument used by those who would equate fetus with person needs to be turned around. Brown argued, for instance, that the burden of proof is on those who say the fetus is not a human person. "We must be able to say we are sure it is *not* human. . . . How can we be sure it is not a human being?"[27] No one can disagree with him that the fetus is human. That is a simple statement that acknowledges the species to which the fetus belongs. Human is an adjective. The fetus is not bovine (cow), or feline (cat), but a *human* conceptus. The problem is asserting that the fetus is a person or human being. The terms are not synonymous. "Human being" is a noun and designates or names a living entity with the qualities of personality and life that

distinguish *Homo sapiens* from all other creatures. Plainly
the presence of life or animation is not a sufficient distinction,
since all animals have life in that sense. The uniqueness of
being person is reflecting the qualities of the image of God.

Furthermore, not every fetus has the potentiality for reflecting the image of God. The abilities of reflective choice,
self-awareness, responsiveness to God and others, and moral
decision-making require some minimum of rational ability
based in biological capacities. When the fetus is spoken of as
being potential person, it is assumed that growth and development are proceeding normally. In cases of radical fetal
deformity the question of potential is not self-evident. Tragically, not all fetuses are conceived with minimal capacities
for personhood. Mistakes are made in nature that leave some
fetuses without a brain or, in some cases, even without recognizable form. Anencephaly, for instance, is a genetic deformity involving only a partial brain or none at all. Such infants
die soon after birth but could be sustained for a longer period
of time. Without a brain one can neither live nor ever develop the unique qualities of personhood. Severe mental
retardation is another case in point, as in trisomy syndrome,
a congenital defect involving an extra thirteenth chromosome. Sixty-five percent of these children die by the third
month, ninety-five percent by three years. All are severely
retarded, continuously hospitalized, and require constant
care. They are in no way able to become persons.

While most people live in splendid isolation from such
cases, the medical profession sees them with sufficient frequency to know that the womb can be a dangerous place.
Cases like these focus the need for legal abortion when couples know they have a fetus that is severely deformed. Anencephaly is detectable early in pregnancy by a relatively simple and inexpensive chemical test for alpha feto proteins.
The same test will detect open spine (spina bifida) and open
skull defects. Trisomy syndrome can be detected by amniocentesis—a pairing of the chromosomes by studying amni-
otic fluid—by the fifteenth week of pregnancy. In cases like

these it is problematic to argue that abortion is the killing of a person. Such fetuses do not have even the potential of growing into what the Bible means by the image of God.

The one who unquestionably fits the biblical portrayal of person is the mother in question. The burden of proof rests with those who would place a fetus on a par with the woman as person. Such an equating fails the test of Scripture and reason. Certainly, the entire circle of those most intimately involved with the abortion question are persons—reflecting on the meaning of this moment, considering the data, weighing the facts of the past, anticipating the future, and making some decision. The abortion question focuses the personhood of the woman, who in turn considers the potential for personhood of the fetus in terms of the multiple dimensions of her own history and the future.

This is a godlike decision for which she is responsible. Like the Creator, she reflects upon what is good for the creation of which she is agent. As steward of those powers, and as co-creator with God, she is to use them for good and not for ill—for herself, the fetus, and the future of humankind itself. She is aware that God wills health and happiness for herself, for those she may bring into the world, and the future of the human race. Thus, she is reflecting on her own well-being, the genetic health of the fetus, and the survival of the human race.

In summary, the biblical perspective on the meaning of personhood focuses on concrete instances of people rather than abstractions like conception or substances that may be infused at conception or during gestation. Nowhere does the Bible settle for a biological definition of personhood. The image of God has no biological equivalent.[28] The Bible does not support the parity argument, since the woman is the obvious concern as person. Furthermore, the language of murder cannot be associated with feticide, or abortion. The Bible does not do so, and those for whom the Bible is truly authoritative will not do so.

Personhood and Moral Responsibility. The New Testa-

ment underscores the responsibility of persons for making
such choices by its emphasis on the priesthood of all believers
(I Peter 2:9), which is an extension and deepening of the Old
Testament idea of *imago Dei* and moral knowledge. Persons
in responsive and responsible relation to the Creator-
Redeemer who is active in their lives and actively involved
in revealing his will to them are here portrayed. The person
not only has direct access to God but has the ability and
responsibility to know and do his will. No other person or
group may arrogate to themselves the right to stand between
the believer and God. Religious imperialism and moralistic
authoritarianism are contradictory to this New Testament
principle.

This points up another important variable in the different
approaches to the abortion question. Those Protestants who
stress the biblical notion of the priesthood of all believers will
be inclined to stress the right and the responsibility of the
woman in making the abortion decision. Those who rely
more on rules and church or religious leader authority models will advocate legal controls. James Gustafson points out
that these arguments are made from an external viewpoint
by people who claim the right to judge the actions of others.
Their model is drawn from the court or the military, deciding
what is right and wrong on the basis of whether it conforms
to certain rules or laws. The data they consider are largely
physical, since they rely on the genetic definition of person.
Finally, their arguments tend to be based on rationalistic
philosophy and natural law which is assumed to be binding
upon all persons in every circumstance and regardless of
their religious persuasion.[29] This is true whether the approach is that of traditional Roman Catholic thought, as in
John Noonan, or in modern evangelicalism, as in Schaeffer
and Brown.

The distinctively Protestant approach focuses upon the
role of the woman rather than upon the abstract notion of life
in the fetus. The great temptation is to act as a moralistic,
external judge who is safely removed from the burden, ter-

ror, and threat of pregnancy. Just as Christians believe that one must experience the truth of the living God before one can truly know what Christian theology is all about, so there is a sense in which only those who experience pregnancy can know what the threat (as well as the joys) of being pregnant is all about. The woman knows uniquely that a pregnancy may cost her her life as well as bring new life into the world. This experiential basis of knowledge is important to moral as well as to religious decision-making. Too often Protestant ethical thought is not true to its own theology which is rooted in grace and love, not law and religious imperialism. As Barth says, Christianity knows "the Word of the free mercy of God which also ascribes and grants freedom to man."[30]

Two factors are important. The first is the experiential basis of religious and moral judgments; the other is the role of conscience in personal moral decision-making. Since men will never experience the threat and terror of childbirth, they are poor arbiters in the debate. Nevertheless, they have been the power brokers, politically, legally, and religiously when it has come to setting the terms for abortion. The abortion question must be dealt with through the eyes of the pregnant woman, not from the safe distance of nonpregnancy or manhood. As Garrett Hardin has noted: "The final straw that breaks the camel's back does not break the legislator's back, nor the theologian's. It breaks hers."[31]

Recovering the biblical notion of the proper role in religion of the individual will shift the debate from "What right does a woman have to an abortion?" to "What right have others to impose an unwanted pregnancy on a woman?" The ethical question is not whether abortion can be justified but whether compulsory pregnancy can be justified.

Sufficient attention has not been given to the moral value of the decision borne and made by the woman whose pregnancy is in question. The spotlight has been focused upon the conceptus as the object of value rather than the woman as moral agent living out the demands of moral freedom and responsibility. Reflecting on why this is the case may lead to endless speculation, of course. One possibility, however, is that what is reflected is the antiwoman bias of so much male-dominated theology. Functionally, the doctrine of "soul competency" (that every individual is directly responsible to God) has served theology better than morals and men better than women. The universality of moral responsibility, however, includes the universality of moral freedom, for in Christ "there is neither male nor female" (Gal. 3:28).

Admittedly, the notion of the soul competency of the believer nurtured among Baptists and others in the free-church tradition tends toward individualism. It stands against the authoritarian or "majority rules" orientation of those traditions more concerned with order and conformity to community expectations. In questions concerning religious freedom from political or ecclesiastical tyranny the doctrine has served to protect private conscience from group tyranny. It also has served to safeguard the right to personal insight into scriptural understandings that may challenge prevailing dogma. Thus, the doctrine has been used theologically and ecclesiastically to safeguard extremely important values.

However, the moral dimensions of soul competency have not been explored sufficiently. Presumably, the fears of moral anarchy or the assumption of clear consensus regarding moral issues have functioned to insist upon moral conformity *and* religious freedom. The question needs to be posed as to whether one does not exclude rather than require the other.

Karl Barth hints at this in his treatment of the moral question of abortion. For him, the primary moral decision is borne by the woman and her physician.[32] Furthermore, the morality of the decision is not determined by the civil law, "because no such law can grasp the fulness of healthy or sick, happy or unhappy, preserved or neglected human life, let alone the freedom of the divine command and the obedience which we owe to it."[33] Precisely because of the fundamental nature of the responsibility involved and the radical obedience that is required, only the woman in question qualifies as the one who may properly respond in freedom and grace. As the pregnancy is hers, so must the moral freedom belong properly to the woman. If the polls are to be believed, a consensus on this matter seems to be developing among Americans in the wake of the Supreme Court decision. This moral understanding is implicit in the theology of soul competency or personal responsibility before God.

Fortunately, this insight is increasingly to be found among Roman Catholics. Bernhard Häring openly challenges the papal ability to settle the question of abortion by invoking the doctrine of infallibility. Häring insists on shared experience and co-reflection where moral matters are concerned. For him, this is necessary because "the final court is the conscience of the physician and/or that of the patient, taking fully into account the doctrine of the magisterium and the endeavors of theologians and other ethicists without which a doctor could not arrive at a thoroughly well informed decision of conscience."[34]

This understanding will also enable us better to understand the absence of a prohibition of abortion in the Bible. Those who are so adamantly determined to prohibit abortion at law have gone to great lengths to find prohibitions in the Bible which are not there. They would not be content unless it explicitly permitted abortion. They like rules for permissible and prohibited behavior, and neither is to be found in the Bible with regard to abortion. Instead, the writers of neither the Old nor the New Testament eras addressed the subject in specific terms. That silence is amazing if, as some contend, the Bible is so clear in its teachings against the practice. We know, for instance, that abortion was practiced in both eras. The harsh laws against women in Semitic areas are evidence that abortion was practiced. Further, the Hebrew law showed the influence of the other Semitic codes. Why was this regulation not included if they were so strongly opposed to it? The silence means either that (1) no Hebrew ever did it and thus no one needed to deal with it; or, (2) the practice was accepted as a family matter and not subject to social regulation. The truth seems to be that it was simply not socially regulated.

Hebrew law gave considerable standing to women in society—which was a primary difference between Hebrew attitudes and those of Assyria, the Hittites, Babylonians, and others. Cultures that gave harsh penalties for abortion were repressive toward women in every area—a fact witnessed even today. Arab girls can still be killed by members of their families for "disgracing" them by marrying a man not approved by the father or by becoming pregnant out of wedlock or by having an abortion.[35] The Hebrews, to the contrary, gave women protection before the law and gave due consideration to their feelings and attitudes in family planning. Rabbi David Feldman, a leading Jewish legal scholar, says that the law sets the well-being of the woman above that of the fetus. If she considers the pregnancy to be a threat to her, she has the support of the law and the community to obtain an abortion. That was and is the dominant Jewish attitude.[36]

This does not mean that the practice was widespread, and we should not conclude that because it was permitted, it was encouraged. It was not. Rabbi Feldman goes on to say that women did not have the moral support of the community if they considered abortion simply for convenience. It was an important decision but by no means a forbidden option.

The same pattern prevailed in New Testament times. The absence of clear references to abortion is amazing, given the context of the Greco-Roman world into which Christianity was born. Of all the vices Paul mentioned in the churches at Rome, Corinth, Thessalonica, Philippi, Ephesus, and Galatia not once did he mention abortion. Those who interpret his condemnation of *pharmakeia* (Gal. 3:1–6; see also Rev. 9:21) as being a prohibition of abortion are pushing the text beyond what it will support. Noonan lamely says that "Paul's usage here cannot be restricted to abortion, but the term he chose is comprehensive enough to include the use of abortifacient drugs."[37]

It is, only if one is determined to find such a prohibition in spite of its absence and if one believes that Paul could not speak clearly. The *pharmakeia* referred to psychogenic drugs used in pagan worship practices. That, as all other practices associated with pagan worship, was forbidden as belonging to the old, that is, pagan way of life. Had Paul felt as strongly about abortion as some modern interpreters say, he would have been very specific, as he was in all matters of interest to him. If ever there was a practical moralist, Paul was. No item escaped his attention as he dealt with guidelines for Christian behavior. The abortion question, however, he left untouched apparently on the basis of the moral principle of Christian freedom. This is an area in which the believer is to "work out your own salvation with fear and trembling; for God is at work in you, both to will and to work for his good pleasure" (Phil. 2:12–13).

Abortion and the Will of God

The Bible holds open the possibility, therefore, that abortion may be consistent with the will of God. Barth understood this in terms of God's "command." For him, the believer knows God's will by "listening" to the revelation of his grace which "is given to us at each moment."[38] This is not a "voice" from God, however, nor is it simply intuition. The believer is first of all attuned to the presence of God in faith —God is actively present in the believer's life. Secondly, one is acquainted with the Scriptures in their totality. Third, one weighs the facts or data. Finally, one discerns personally the "command" of God.

Barth's treatment of abortion is set in the context of "the protection of life." He first explored "the great summons to halt issued by the command" forbidding the willful taking of human life.[39] The first step is to hear God's "No!" to any such action. Barth emphatically warned of the danger in ever considering the possibility that killing may be either permissible or necessary regardless of circumstances. He recognized that notions of the exceptional case run the risk of reflecting arbitrary desires or self-justification. These temptations must be avoided. Thus, Barth begins with a presumption in favor of keeping alive, or no abortion.

However, he also perceived the "other side" of God's command. Having heard the command against terminating life, he says, we must be "prepared . . . to stand by the truth that at some time or other, perhaps on the far frontier of all other possibilities, it may have to happen in obedience to the commandment that men must be killed by men."[40] The unborn cannot claim to be preserved in all circumstances. God may call for the active participation of people in the killing of germinating life.[41] When he does so, it does not constitute murder.

Care must be taken, of course, to spell out the narrow parameters in which abortion may be understood as the command of God. Stress must be placed on the tentative nature or the substantive mood in which it is made. *May be* understood does not mean *is* or *must be* understood. The command of God to abort is a secondary command to that of keeping alive. "Secondary" does not mean less important, however, but more nearly means "less frequently given." This is both a religious and a practical understanding: practical in that, as long as the desires of nature are intact concerning sexual congress, and the protective dynamics of the desirability of children, population growth stability, and symbiotic mother-conceptus relationships are functional, the widespread incidence of conception and birth (i.e., the command to procreate) will be assured. In addition, the requirements of conscience on the part of those who feel strongly about abortion will serve as adequate constraint on the practice.

Even so, the secondary command "to abort" will also be heard by significant numbers of persons. Among these certainly will be women with unwanted pregnancies who hear the command to terminate. Included also will be that coterie of persons who support her decision and empathetically live the experience—family, the health care team, social scientists, philosophers, ethicists, theologians, and others.

Barth was struggling with the problem of the rightness of an action in the exceptional case. He saw clearly that if any act is permitted by God or is related positively to the will of God, the act is morally right. It was not "the lesser of two evils" or unforgivable sin. Barth used the designation "the command of God" for this morally proper and correct, even if socially suspect or legally prohibited, act.

Procreation and the Control of Fertility. To be sure, the tension between the command to procreate and the command to terminate must be maintained. However, the command to procreate is much more easily heard than the command to terminate. The sexual drive is a powerful urge that has ensured the proliferation of the species. Theologically, this natural urge has been interpreted as the command of God to "be fruitful and multiply, and fill the earth" (Gen. 1:28). Understandably, the religious focus for centuries in the life of the people of God was upon procreation. There was a need for people. That need was rooted in the need for human survival itself.

The command to procreate may be understood as the divine will that the human species should be perpetuated. This noble experiment of the divine activity should not perish from the face of the earth. God willed that people should live because of the unique features of humanness itself. This helps to focus the problem of hearing the command of God to terminate embryonic life. Hearing the command is rooted in self-transcendence—the person's capacity to understand the processes of which he or she is a part. People are able to analyze cause-and-effect relationships and to govern—to "have dominion over" (Gen. 1:28b)—the processes in which they are involved. The creation narratives plainly envision people as comprehending the divine command as purposeful and directed activity. For this reason, procreation for people was different than for the rest of the created order. All animal life multiplies. All living organisms perpetuate their own kind. This is the divine will (Gen. 1:20–24).

However, only people have the capacity to govern the

process, for only they comprehend the relationship between sexual congress and procreation. This is why the necessity for controlling birth is a logical (and theological) corollary to humanity's realization of the necessity for procreation. Human rational powers are no less related to and subject to obey the divine command than are genital powers. For people to hear only the command to procreate is to deny the essence of human uniqueness—the ability to participate with discriminating understanding in the creative activity of God.

Just as people hear the command to propagate, they also must hear the command to control their fertility. Abortion may at times be understood as the command to control population growth. Procreation is both promise and threat, first to the woman, then to society itself. It promises the perpetuation of the species and threatens the species with destruction or extinction. Thus, the command to survive is also the command to limit growth.

This recognition is in part related to our "coming of age" with regard to the medical revolution. While "hearing" the command of God to "keep alive," people have inadvertently failed to notice that life-threatening circumstances are being created. Increasingly, both science and theology are realizing that the benefits of medical advances cannot be accepted without our bearing the anxieties and consequences of its responsibilities. We are often blind to the larger social costs exacted by biomedical advances.

The signs of the times bear an ominous message: limited resources can support only a limited population. In terms of available resources, earth is apparently already vastly overpopulated. The future seems destined for an increasingly desperate battle for the survival of masses of people where the birth of children is greeted as sad tragedy and the circumstances of life are more nearly described as death.

The more abundant the population grows, the more desperate the circumstances of living become and the less valuable individual life becomes. Life is reduced to "nature, red in tooth and claw" in the mad scramble for life-sustaining resources. The Ik, a tribe of northern Uganda, may be such a sign. Their numbers exceed their resources, so that each person pits skills and wit to survive against others. Children are put out of the home at the age of three and no one shares any morsel of food or moment of compassion with another. An anthropologist commented that they have lost their humanness and that, as a people, they are passing into extinction.

Surely it is not too much to imagine that, in retrospect, measures to control population growth were *required* in order to assure the survival of this people. The larger issue of overpopulation on a worldwide scale cannot be isolated from the specific matter of human conception. In its larger frame of reference, therefore, the so-called "tragedy" of abortion may well be a requirement of human survival. Too many modern ills are created by the refusal to set particular issues in their larger contexts.

The notion that controlling human fertility is morally wrong is unbiblical, antilife, and antihuman. Such teaching is not based on the Bible. However, it condemns those simple but faithful followers of that teaching to an endless cycle of poverty and malnutrition. Large portions of the human race suffer as nature moves to redress the balance.

Population will be controlled—at least to some extent. The question is the manner in which it is controlled. Either people will take steps to control growth by measures worthy of human personalities or they will be controlled by forces that deny the worth and dignity of those personalities. Those forces are "red in tooth and claw." Famine, war, pestilence, and disease are the terrible front four of inhumane ways of controlling swarming hordes of people on earth. Poverty, malnourishment, brain disease, and social disorder are the four antihuman legacies of a theology that rules against "artificial" means and in favor of "nature's way."

The will of God is that people be good stewards of all their powers—sexual, rational, and spiritual. Those who do not exercise constraint in the number of children they bear are faithless stewards denying the dignity with which and for which people have been created. Such an ethic violates the command of God to be good stewards of sexual powers. God wills that the human race be blessed and not cursed by progeny. The promise of God is that his people should live long upon the earth. But uncontrolled fertility threatens that future and the realization of God's promise.

The moral need for fertility control is not based simply on consequentialist calculations of how population growth threatens the human race. The threat is there and can be perceived. But these are signs that underscore the moral requirement of God's will regarding human sexuality from the beginning.

Every act of coitus should not be open to the possibility of conception. Far from it. Coitus should be an act of responsible stewardship. The biblical command to "be fruitful, and multiply, and replenish the earth" (Gen. 1:28) has a crucial qualifier. "Replenish" does not mean "fill" but "replace what is lost" or "provide what is needed." The command is not to overpopulate but to adequately populate. Those who emphasize the "be fruitful and multiply" without the qualifier distort the meaning of this command. The result is a demonic inversion of the divine intention.

The procreative purpose of sex is of secondary or even tertiary importance in the Bible. The oldest creation account is found in Genesis 2. It emphasizes the companionate purpose of marriage. Male and female are brought to union for affection and companionship. People are social creatures; their need for one another is by the creative will of God. The writer declared that God created male and female, for it was "not good that the man should be alone." Sexuality was created to serve the human need for companionship and intimacy. The consummation of this union was that "they become one flesh" (Gen. 2:24). No procreative purpose is involved here; children are not mentioned.[42]

The importance of this passage is that it establishes the priority or primacy of purposes regarding sexuality in the

Hebrew mind. This passage is not of most importance just because it is older. It is older because it is of most importance. The passage concerning procreation (Gen. 1:27) is later and points to one of the important, but not the most important, purposes of sexual intercourse.

We can see this order of importance by observing the place of sexuality in human life. People need the intimacy of sexual intercourse entirely apart from the need for children. Whether or not children are either wanted or needed to "replenish the earth," people need the benefits of intimacy, caring, and comfort that are derived from coitus. Were the natural law theorists consistent in their logic, procreation would not be the primary purpose of coitus. The problem is that their norm was derived from a combination of Stoic philosophy stressing divine reason and a study of "the laws of nature" at work among animals other than people. The animals of the field are dominated by sex related to the oestrus season of the female.[43]

With few exceptions, animals engage in sexual intercourse for procreation. Adopting that as a moral norm for people, however, is problematic. The proper study of man is man, declared Alexander Pope in an obvious criticism of those who attempt to govern people by norms derived from other species. This is another sign of the antihuman bias of a natural law sexual ethic.

The mischief and misery created by this moral tradition are a result of failure to follow the teachings of Scripture. Biblical perspectives were replaced by philosophical norms. These attitudes were then imposed upon the Bible, as filters through which the Bible was interpreted. Tradition and the theology of the church were used to interpret the Bible. Biblical authority was replaced by the authority of the church.

That turn was tragic and has left faithful Christians with a misguided and destructive ethic instead of the biblical ethic intended to bless and preserve the human race. The recognition of biblical authority instead of a bending toward philosophical traditions will be a necessary first step in the recovering of a perspective regarding human sexuality that leads to the wholeness of persons and the preservation of the human race.

With regard to abortion, this has two meanings. Negatively, it means that an insistence on the supreme value and complete rights of every particular conceptus may destroy the very goal being sought, namely, the perpetuation of the human race. Positively, it means that an abortion may be a particular response to the command of God to preserve the human race. To those who hear that command, the religious community should give the full support of its redemptive ministry.

The Grace and Providence of God. A final factor in discerning the will of God involves the way in which God is related to the entire process of conception and birth or the processes of nature. Some people argue that God has directly willed every conception regardless of the circumstances. Thus, to terminate a pregnancy is to contradict "what God has done." This poses the question as to the nature of God in his providential care for his children.

Donald Shoemaker, for instance, argues that abortion is forbidden in cases of rape. He gives a *non sequitur* about not executing the rapist for the crime and asks rhetorically if we then are to mete out capital punishment upon the innocent unborn? His clinching argument, however, is "God forbid that we should regard any situation as so tragic that God could not have prevented it if he so chose." He proceeds to apply this same logic to cases of incest and fetal deformity.[44]

In effect, Shoemaker is arguing that God is responsible for the pregnancy by rape. God wills the pregnancy, for "he could have prevented it." Logically, he would also have to argue that God willed the rape since that "could have been prevented" and since the rape was necessary for the impregnation. He counsels those women who have been so victimized to look for some hidden purpose of God behind the seeming tragedy. He piously dodges the issue of dealing with the nature of evil by declaring: "God makes no mistakes."

Applied to the issue of impregnation by rape, Shoemaker's theology poses profound questions. He seems to believe that God causes such tragedies to teach stern lessons to his children. The comfort he offers the woman impregnated by rape is that "no testing will overtake one except those God has permitted men [sic!] to experience."[45]

Here is a stress on the sovereignty of God that combines theological ideas of the power and activity of God with a type of "law of nature's way." This is similar to but without the sophistication of natural law theory. The "causal connection between sexual intercourse and conception . . . is simply the means whereby God, the first cause of all things, gives his blessing."[46] In other words, God causes whatever happens in nature.

This view of the working of God in nature and history is certainly not new. But it is dealt with in the Bible and emphatically rejected from Job to Jesus. This overemphasizes the power of God while compromising the goodness of God. To argue seriously that God either causes directly or permits rape or incest and consequent pregnancy is to say heretical and blasphemous things about God.

Central to the teaching of Jesus was the idea that God is love and goodness. He emphatically denounced and refuted the theology that God caused evil things to happen to people. He drew a very simple test for knowing whether God would do a certain thing: "If you . . . , who are evil, know how to give good gifts to your children, how much more will your Father who is in heaven give good things to those who ask him!" (Matt. 7:11). Being able to rely on the goodness of God was central to Jesus' teaching about prayer (Luke 12), and God as loving Father is the all-pervasive notion of God's character that appears in the parables of Jesus.

Apparently some people would rather portray God as cruel and capricious than admit he may not be totally in control of every event. However, Jesus took a dim view of people crediting good acts to the evil one and evil acts to

God. That confuses the work of the Creator-Redeemer with that of the adversary (see Matt. 12:22–32; Luke 11:14–23). God does not cause women to be raped or children to be incestuously impregnated. In such events, people are confronted with the sin of man. In the face of the recalcitrant and rebellious will of men, God is powerless to intervene (Luke 15:11–32). God grants freedom to individuals—even the freedom to sin in ways that injure and destroy God's creation and other creatures. Murder, rape, and mayhem all belong to the human story of sinful rebellion from the will of the Creator. God is not the author of sin, nor the source of the temptation to violate another person's integrity (see James 1:13–15).

Another problem posed by Shoemaker's approach is its limited and inadequate view of the grace of God. He declares that God gives "sustaining grace" to those afflicted with pregnancy by rape or incest or those who bear fetuses which are radically deformed. To be sure, God does offer the strength of his Spirit for those difficult and unavoidable cases. But his grace also gives permission to act in spite of ambiguity and tragedy. The last word in the history of God's revelation was not Sinai but Calvary and Easter. With boldness, Christians lay hold of God's promise of forgiveness in their struggle against the evils they confront. The paradox of God's willing both the protection of germinating life and its destruction under certain circumstances is at the heart of the biblical message and a necessary part of the meaning of the grace of God in the tragic circumstances of life.

It is not the will of God that any woman be impregnated by rape, nor by incest. To insist that women must remain pregnant under such circumstances is to take sides with the evil against which we must all struggle. The ethical principle is that pregnancy should be by choice and not by compulsion.[47] The woman is doubly victimized when she is compelled to bear a pregnancy by rape or incest—first by the man who violated her body and her moral integrity and second by a society that violates her freedom to act out her conscientious stewardship before God. The grace of God is available to those facing such choices and is sufficient to provide wisdom and sustaining strength. Legal constraints based on narrow religious moralisms ought not frustrate the work of God, who is working for the redemption of the woman in the midst of sinful and evil circumstances.

CONCLUSION

The Bible gives a great deal of guidance on the abortion issue. This is not in the form of a rule or commandment prohibiting abortion, nor even casuistic details regarding circumstances under which it may be permitted or prohibited. It is neither prohibited nor prescribed. Rather, perspectives are given on each of the critical factors in such a way that the believer may render a faithful response following the leadership of God's Spirit.

In terms of the current debate, the claim that the Bible teaches that the fetus is a person from the moment of conception has been tested and found wanting. This notion is from natural law theory, not from the Bible. The biblical portrait of person is focused in the man and woman who unquestionably bear the image of God, who stand directly responsible to God, and who are called to render a faithful stewardship of procreative powers before God. Stewardship involves accepting the role of co-creator with God, responsibly controlling human fertility, and making decisions regarding the circumstances under which God would have couples bring children into the world.

Further, the Bible gives no support for those efforts to prohibit abortion at law. It is clearly not "antiabortion" in the sense that contemporary groups would have us believe. Certainly, fetal life is to be taken with radical seriousness, but it is not to be given ultimate standing or even equal standing with the woman before the law. The silence of the Bible on the subject of elective abortion is an eloquent testimony to the sacredness of this choice for women and their families and the privacy in which it is to be considered. Those who follow the Bible will resist efforts to make this intensely personal and private choice a matter for public ridicule or regulation.

Finally, the Bible makes it clear that the last word in the abortion decision is not one of guilt but of forgiveness. In the midst of the moral ambiguity of tragic and perplexing circumstances, God gives grace and direction. Strength will be provided for one to decide and follow on the basis of one's religious understandings, moral convictions, and personal circumstances. One is free to abort or not to abort, as God leads. This is the freedom of grace.

Chapter 4

EUTHANASIA:
THE PERSON AND DEATH

Is the notion of "death with dignity" in any way supportable on biblical grounds? Does one have a moral right to "die well" or experience a "good death" that is rooted in Christian theology? May one actually aid the coming of death or choose the manner of one's dying, or is death strictly within the province of God?

Questions like these point to the moral dilemmas related both to elective death—a type of suicide—and to what is popularly referred to as euthanasia, or mercy killing. The debate between those who support and those who oppose the notion of elective death has generated an intensity almost equal to that regarding abortion. Linkage between the basic assumptions of the opposing groups is acknowledged by both sides, but such strong passions are evoked that little discussion of the underlying theological issues takes place. What is at stake is no less than competing attitudes toward the proper role of persons regarding choosing or resisting death.

FACING THE ISSUES

The moral issues regarding elective death may be focused around two cases that have gained widespread attention in both religious and secular circles. The first is that of Karen Ann Quinlan of New Jersey, who has been comatose since

April 15, 1975. She had collapsed after a party during which she had ingested both alcoholic beverages and drugs. She was entered into the hospital after being resuscitated twice—first by friends and then by the emergency ambulance crew. For the next fourteen months she was kept continuously on a respirator.

Her medical condition is described as one of a "persistent vegetative state." She has irreversible brain damage, no cognitive or cerebral functioning, and virtually no chance for any return of discriminating ability. During hospitalization, her body has deteriorated to less than seventy pounds weight. The cause of her condition is a lesion of the cerebral hemisphere and a lesion in the brain stem. She remains in coma even through the respirator has been removed.

By now the Quinlan name is virtually a household word in America because the plight of her parents has been followed by the news media. Dedicated Roman Catholics, they took the case to court to seek the legal guardianship of Karen and to obtain explicit authority to order the discontinuance of the artificial respirator. That request was denied by Superior Court Judge Robert Muir, Jr., but affirmed by the Supreme Court of New Jersey. By that time, however, Karen began to breathe on her own, much to the amazement of her doctors. Apparently, her heart began to function without the normal neurological support system of the brain. She now is cared for in a New Jersey nursing home, where she is fed intravenously but without hope of recovery.

The second case is that of Dr. and Mrs. Henry P. van Dusen. Dr. Van Dusen was an internationally known and highly respected theologian and past president of Union Theological Seminary in New York City. In January 1975, the Van Dusens took an overdose of sleeping pills in a covenant to commit suicide. She died from the overdose, he regurgitated the pills and was hospitalized. Three weeks later he died of a heart attack. Mrs. Van Dusen was eighty years of age and was lame from advanced arthritis which confined her to a wheelchair. He was seventy-seven, had suffered repeated strokes which left him unable to communicate normally or be active. Their decision to die was prompted by the fact that they could only anticipate continued physical and mental deterioration to the point of complete helplessness or total dependency on life-maintaining machines. They decided to terminate living under their present circumstances and thus have some measure of control over the manner of death.

These cases focus important issues for public and private discussions regarding death and dying. The Quinlan case raises the issue of *the manner in which one may die.* The options or possibilities are many, of course. Death may happen suddenly as a result of an accident or a heart attack. Or it may occur more slowly from a lingering illness. One may die peacefully or after months or even years of pain and suffering. There is little way to know how death will happen. Increasingly, however, the prospects are that one will die after an extensive process of wasting away, or that death will come only after the extensive and exhaustive ministrations of medical science have been applied. The art of caring for the dying during their final days is increasingly being turned into a science of postponing death. Karen Ann Quinlan is a symbol of a new anxiety introduced into the sociology of medicine. That is the ever-present fear of artificially supported life well beyond the point of natural death. A new image of death has entered the ranks of those already entertained by people who reflect upon the inevitability of death. That is death after months of coma or unconsciousness sustained by an efficient but uncaring machine while one vital organ after another deteriorates.

The peaceful deathbed scene with family gathered for the last moment together is becoming a thing of the past. Jacob anticipated and prepared for his imminent death by calling his sons together and spoke a final, personal word with each of them. Lucid and communicative, he spoke with unimpaired insight into the character of each son. He also gave detailed instructions for his burial, clarifying the title to his family burial plot. His death came gently: "When Jacob finished charging his sons, he drew up his feet into the bed, and breathed his last, and was gathered to his people" (Gen. 49:33).

Such scenes are now more nostalgic relics of the past than possibilities for the future. Death now comes in hospitals, and more than likely is separated from friends and family. The patient is more likely to be unconscious than communicative, expiring after desperate efforts to prolong vital life signs—a scene of suspended bottles, plastic tubes, and intricate life-sustaining equipment. Medical technology has contributed to greater longevity and created a new mysticism as to its powers to prolong life. Death cannot be defeated but it can be delayed. But only at enormous cost, perhaps the greatest of which is the tragic depersonalization of life sustained artificially with no prospect of cure. Karen Quinlan has become an ominous and perhaps tragic sign of medical technology and of our personal future.

No one wants to die like that. This is not motivated by a preoccupation with pain or a narcissistic concern about appearance but by a concern for the person as person.[1] Subjected to procedures over which one has no say and reduced to an object of medical manipulation, the person as person usually disappears long before the machines are turned off and death is pronounced. As Häring says, "It is pitiful to see how persons in modern, well-equipped hospitals are manipulated by a whole system of machinery and activity, not for healing but only for prolonging the coma."[2]

While it may be difficult to anticipate those circumstances under which one would want a respirator turned off, it is not difficult to anticipate *that* one may want it removed. In the light of such prospects, some have refused to enter hospitals during the last stages of terminal illness. Senator Wayne Morse refused dialysis when his kidneys failed. Colonel Charles Lindbergh, after accepting treatment in the early stages of terminal cancer, retreated to the island of Maui and there made preparation to die. These persons decided to resist the encroachment of medical technology on their individual personhood. Many have applauded their decision as heroic and symbolically important. Ramsey, commenting on the human will to resist technological take-overs at one's dying, wrote: "Rather than remain the purely passive patient of spectacular medical powers, he may stick out his tongue at the idea . . . and *freely and responsibly choose to die.*"[3]

This also raises a moral question for the medical profession itself since the medical technologist, armed with sophisticated tools of science, may be extremely hard to get away from once one enters the hospital. Before the advent of death-delaying devices, a person died once—at home or office or in the field. Now one may die several times, as resuscitative measures are repeatedly employed to restore "life after death." Since science is better able to keep alive than to heal the terminally ill,[4] the question must be posed as to the morally legitimate limits of interfering with dying which may be more akin to torture than to therapy. Certainly, respect for the dying life as such forbids an unnecessary and unwarranted torturing even in the name of medical procedure.[5]

The second issue raised by these cases concerns the *right to decide, within limits, the circumstances under which one dies.* The issue is not whether or not one may decide to die! Death has an exceptionally high batting average. The fact that people die is an axiom of existence. The question is whether or not one has a right to decide the terms for death or the circumstances under which death will be experienced. The Van Dusens, for instance, decided to die from an overdose of barbiturates rather than wait until their physical and mental condition had so deteriorated that they would have no control over their dying or living. While they were able, they decided to set the terms under which death would come to them.

The Van Dusens are not alone in believing that one should be able to participate in the death decision. Suicide under similar circumstances is not at all uncommon. The writings of Ernest Hemingway reflected a philosophical concern for the meaning of death and the person's approach to dying. His heroes were men who, knowing that death (or tragedy) was going to overtake them, exerted their will in order to set the terms on which it happened. The ability to set the terms with death—which involved both a calculation about and an anticipation of death and the determination to carry out the scheme—was based on uniquely human capacities. For Hemingway, the person was "defined" by his ability to face defeat in a heroic way. His own death testified to the depth of that conviction. Suffering from recurrent bouts with psychosis, he anticipated the approach of both mental incapacity and death under those circumstances—eventually. He chose another route. In one of his lucid moments, he killed himself with a shotgun.[6]

Lael Wertenbaker wrote of her husband's experience with cancer. Before going into the last stages of his illness, which would have included coma, incapacity, and unrelievable pain, he decided to set the terms for his death. After an overdose of drugs failed to do more than make him nauseated, he slashed his wrists and died in the presence of his faithful wife, who had supported him during his ordeal.[7]

The moral question raised by stories like these is whether or not such actions violate something profoundly human or tend to destroy personal values in such a way that they can only be regarded as immoral or sinful. Are such suicides a violation of the will of God and his commandment, "You shall not kill" (Ex. 20:13)? Or can it be argued that we should be able to participate in our own dying by deciding the manner of death? Might such an act be one of faith and consistent with biblical understandings of human responsibility before God?

There is still a third question involved in the contemporary debates about euthanasia which is posed by cases such as those of infants or the terminally ill who are dying. The issue concerns the morality of mercy in aiding the dying patient. The question goes beyond simply withdrawing treatments.

The issue is whether, in the name of mercy, one might morally aid someone's dying? Are there circumstances under which it is morally responsible actively to terminate a person, or does love always require resisting death through every means possible? Fletcher declares bluntly that "it is harder morally to justify letting somebody die a slow and ugly death, dehumanized, than it is to justify helping him to escape from such misery."[8]

This is more than an abstract problem of interest to philosophers and theologians. Some very prominent people are making pacts with friends or relatives that specify that either will help the other die when life becomes desperate from pain or tragic accident. Dr. Christiaan Barnard, famous heart surgeon from South Africa, has entered such an agreement with his brother, who is also a physician.

Families and physicians feel a variety of powerful emotions when dealing with a patient dying a slow and agonizing death. Certainly they wish the pain relieved and health restored; that the patient not die but go on living and sharing concerns and joys together. When the illness is terminal and there is no hope of relief or recovery, however, death is often desired for the patient as God's appointed way to relieve suffering. One woman shared her experience at the death of her husband after his prolonged battle with cancer. He had deteriorated physically and mentally practically beyond recognition. "I prayed for death," she said, "because I loved him and could not bear to see him suffer so. And when death finally came, I thanked God for his good gift."

But suppose her husband had asked her to help him die! She felt already that death was imminent and desirable. As a Christian she felt that death would be a merciful relief of pain and suffering. Could she have been morally justified to act out her love for him by ending his suffering in some painless manner?

A physician at one of the leading hospitals in the South described his feelings when his own mother was dying of cancer. He felt she should have been relieved of her pain, though no drug was available that would not also bring death. He found himself wishing that someone would help her die, and was suddenly caught up in a struggle of conscience. Knowing what *could* be done and wanting to relieve her suffering, he faced the moral dilemma of whether in fact to help her die. At that point, he said, he retreated from her room so as not to watch her agony. He confessed relief when she finally died. When he was asked why he did not aid her dying, his answer was that he was not sure he could have lived with his conscience if he had. He did not feel it would have been wrong, only that he could not live with it.

His dilemma as a Christian physician is increasingly commonplace. Does mercy for the dying require more than active efforts to keep alive or passively allow them to die? Must death be actively resisted or passively awaited, or might it be actively invited? The answers one gives to these questions will depend upon a variety of assumptions regarding the meaning of death, the morality of taking or ending life—one's own or another's—and the relationship of the person to the processes of nature and the activity of God in one's life.

EUTHANASIA: ANCIENT AND MODERN

The concern to die well is as old as humanity itself, for the questions surrounding death belong to the essence of being human. All creatures die, but apparently only people know they are to die. They live with the axiom that life is under the sentence of death. That knowledge adds a dimension to human life that has no parallel in the rest of creation. Anxiety about death and the threat of annihilation are universal experiences among people. People are products of nature and the natural processes. They are intimately and dependently bound to nature but are able to transcend it through thought and self-conscious, deliberate action. All relations toward death are in this situation of strength and weakness—dominion and dependency.[9] Thus, from the beginning of the species concern with how one dies has been an implicit part of the human attempt to come to terms with death.

The term "euthanasia" means "good death" or "well dying"; it is derived from the Greek *eu* and *thanatos*. In its classical sense, it is a descriptive term referring to an easy death as opposed to an agonizing or tormented dying. In Greek literature euthanasia connoted a "happy death, an ideal and coveted end to a full and pleasant life."[10] Among the Romans a similar meaning was preserved. As Suetonius wrote of the death of Caesar Augustus: "He expired suddenly . . . dying a very easy death, and much as he himself had always wished for." The Stoics, such as Seneca, used the term to refer to a "noble" death, which they regarded as a fitting climax to a valiant life, and an ever-available route of escape from living under intolerable circumstances. To be sure, their glowing estimate of the glory of death was premised on their philosophies of the immortality of the soul. But their acceptance of death as an end to be acknowledged, for which preparation is to be made and which is not an ultimate threat to human well-being, is a point in common with Jewish and Christian understandings.

The ease of Jacob's death was typical of a desirable ending to human life among Jews. After a gratifying life and as he came to the fullness of years, he was "gathered to his people." Abraham was promised that he would go to his fathers in peace and "be buried in a good old age" (Gen. 15:15). Isaac died peacefully (Gen. 35:29), as did Gideon (Judg. 8:32), David (I Chron. 29:28), Jehoiada (II Chron. 24:15), and Job (Job 42:17). No tragedy was attached to death as long as there had been a normal life span, one had children for posterity, and no scandal would forbid burial with honor.[11] This latter concern was a point of distress for Jesus and his interpreters in coming to grips with the scandal of the cross (Matt. 26:36–46; I Cor. 1:23). However, Christ transformed even the meaning of the cross. It became a sign of assurance and hope as Christians confronted death. Paul's reflection on the matter summarized this insight: "Whether we live or whether we die, we are the Lord's" (Rom. 14:8). The concern had been shifted from the manner in which one died, to the purpose for which one lived. Death, regardless of how it came to one who lived righteously before God, was a good death.

To die well one must therefore live well. Preparation for the encounter with death is necessary if one is not to be unduly anxious about it or be destroyed by fear. This was the concern of the *ars moriendi* that developed in the Middle Ages. Knowing that death is inevitable and anticipating one's own experience required cultivating the art of dying well.

The moral acceptability of suicide has been debated among philosophers from Pythagoras to Camus. Many argued that suicide was immoral. Pythagoras' objection was religious—without God's command one has no right to kill God's property. Plato said it was the person's duty to stay alive for service, and Aristotle objected on the ground of civic obligation.

The Stoics generally accepted suicide as a cure for life's burdens. Hegesias presented such appealing arguments that he was forbidden to lecture on the subject. Some moved from approving it under exceptionable circumstances to making it a duty should one conclude death was advisable. The Epicureans regarded death as an evil but acknowledged that suicide was acceptable when life became an even greater evil. On the island of Cos, the birthplace of Hippocrates, there was a custom for old men who had grown weary of life to drink hemlock together.

Some Christian writers, such as Jerome, approved of suicide in defense of virginity, though most argued that it hindered the soul's passage into eternity. The Council of Arles condemned suicide as inspired by Satan. Aquinas formulated the teaching still held by orthodox Roman Catholics. His arguments added the notion that suicide violates the Sixth Commandment to those objections already registered by Plato, Aristotle, and the Neoplatonists. He added gravity to their objections by saying it precluded forgiveness and thus incurred eternal punishment.

Sir Thomas More advocated voluntary euthanasia for those suffering from incurable and painful disease. Francis Bacon, a century later, argued that doctors should assist those who wish to die. For him, the physician's duty was "to mitigate pains and dolors, and not only when such mitigation may conduce to recovery, but when it may serve to make a faire and easy passage."

John Donne, claiming that suicide was not inherently evil, defended it under certain circumstances on the grounds of Christian theology. Published posthumously, the work was entitled *Biathanatos*.[12] David Hume's 1757 essay "On Suicide" argued that a person had a "native liberty" to determine his death under certain circumstances such as pain and disease. He skillfully refuted the main religious objections, saying it was not necessarily sin.

Kant argued that suicide contradicted the categorical imperative, but his philosophical argument on the whole could be used to support its acceptability. Nietszche rejected suicide, saying that one ought to assert one's will against all pain and suffering. Even so, because of his bad health, he often took overdoses of chloral, hoping to die. He also admitted that contemplating suicide helped him get through many a bad night. Jeremy Bentham accepted the notion of suicide on utilitarian grounds or the pleasure-pain principle and demanded assistance in his dying moments. William James rejected suicide at the theoretical level on pragmatic grounds, but suffered bouts of suicidal depression and admitted that probably every educated person had considered suicide. Freud explained suicide as the death wish in immature people but died at his request for a lethal injection to end his pain from cancer of the jaw.

Albert Camus regarded suicide as the only serious philosophical problem stemming from his notion that life was absurd. He held that suicide acknowledges that life is not worth the trouble.[13] Even so, he did not recommend suicide but that people discover meaning by becoming involved with suffering humanity.

This brief summary of the debate in historical perspective makes several things obvious. First, there have been strong differences of opinion among people of goodwill, profound religious faith, and unquestioned intelligence. Second, the different moral judgments reflected varying assumptions about death, the nature of God, salvation and the afterlife, the role of reason and the meaning of life. Third, in general, those who oppose suicide do so on the basis of one or more moral principles, while those who make some allowance for suicide move to ground-of-meaning considerations.[14] Thus, Aquinas uses the commandment against murder, Plato the principle of duty, and Kant the "formal rule" of the categorical imperative. On the other hand, the Stoics appealed to the freedom and immortality of the soul, Donne focused on the question of evil, Hume on human rights and anthropology, and Camus on the meaning of life. The use of principles can also be seen in justifying suicide by writers like Francis Bacon, who stressed the principle of the duty to relieve pain and assist the dying. A final characteristic is that, among those who give any approval to suicide, there are limits or constraints around the types of suicide considered. While many oppose suicide for any reason or under any circumstances, most who approve it do so only under certain conditions, usually the imminence of death.

Similar grounds for argument can be found in the contemporary debate. Neither theological and philosophical questions nor the principles felt to be appropriate have been radically altered. What has changed is the situation or circumstances under which death might be experienced, namely, advanced medical technology. To the anxieties produced by the prospect of painful death is now added the anxiety of being unable to escape the use of sophisticated machines. There are, therefore, new moral issues. These include the right of the patient to refuse treatment, the morality of prolonging the dying process after sentient life has passed or there is no reasonable prospect for meaningful recovery, and whether medical knowledge should be used to hasten death in the terminally ill and unconscious patient.

The parameters of the discussion do not include what has been called "compulsory euthanasia" such as was used in Hitler's death camps.[15] Popular associations of euthanasia with the Nazi atrocities are both misleading and inaccurate. Those who oppose any form of euthanasia frequently make such allegations in a guilt-by-association tactic. There is no justification for arguing, however, that the *first* use of the term "euthanasia" was in Germany in 1920, which then became the rationale behind Nazi genocide.[16]

The unfortunate consequence of such arguments is the clouding of the legitimate issues at stake in the debate about medical technology and its relation to human dying.[17] Hitler's gas chambers were not merciful but merciless; killing was by political coercion, not voluntary consent; and the patients were not dying but, for ideological reasons, were judged undesirable. This does not mean that the Nazi use of medicine for political purposes has no bearing on a discussion of the ethical uses of medicine. Plainly it does. That tragic era stands as a grim reminder of the dangers of permitting medical practice to come under political control and of the legitimate moral limits of using medicine to bring about death.

Two primary factors set the limits of the current debate. One is the imminence of death and the other is patient consent. Euthanasia deals with the terms under which or the manner in which one is to die when death is already imminent. Fletcher defines it as "the deliberate easing into death of a patient suffering from a painful and fatal disease."[18] There is a vital moral difference between (1) putting to death certain categories of people who are otherwise healthy; and (2) helping someone die out of mercy when it is known they are dying or they are hopelessly beyond the point of recovering personal wholeness.

TYPES OF ELECTIVE DEATH

There are three interrelated sets of factors where death decisions are concerned. One is the type of action that might be taken, another concerns the consent or request of the patient, and the third is the means employed. These are so interrelated that at least six typologies can be distinguished.

1. The first is *active, voluntary, and indirect.* This is not, properly speaking, a form of euthanasia, but it deserves mention in this context as a matter of clarification and distinction. Senator Wayne Morse and Colonel Charles Lindbergh were mentioned as having refused medical treatment knowing they had an incurable illness. Their decision was voluntary and was actively carried out by them, but death came indirectly—by disease.

2. The second is *active, voluntary, and direct.* The patient makes the death decision and carries it out, using direct means. This is also called euthanatic suicide and involves actions such as those of the Van Dusens and Wertenbaker. The most familiar and least shocking type is that in which the patient takes an overdose of medicine. This is widely regarded as a type of rational suicide.[19] That is, the patient is not mentally ill or incompetent. The person acts on the basis of personal freedom and in the light of attitudes toward what it means to live and when it is desirable to die. Groups such as Society for the Right to Die, and Exit, in Britain, are founded on the philosophy that each person has a basic, human right to make such a decision and take such action freely.

3. A third type is *passive, voluntary, and direct.* The patient exacts a pledge from someone else—friend, relative, physician—to hasten his dying or to intervene to bring death more quickly if he is unable to do it himself.[20] The agreement may be made well in advance of the problem or once the patient is already infirm. This is the type of covenant the Barnard brothers have entered into.

This places great moral responsibility, mental burden, and legal vulnerability upon those who enter such a covenant. The act, however, is the carrying out of a promise made to the patient and under circumstances set by the patient himself. The moral rightness of the commitment to mercifully foreshorten pain is seen as the justification for the tragedy involved in terminating life. Sometime ago national attention was drawn to a New Jersey case involving Lester Zygmaniak, who killed his brother in a hospital. George, 26, had been paralyzed from his neck down as a result of a motorcycle accident. Because both brothers had been active outdoorsmen, they had agreed to be killed by the other should either become incapacitated. Lester shot George with a shotgun, was tried for homicide, but was acquitted.[21]

4. The fourth type is *passive, voluntary, and indirect.*[22] It differs from the third type only in the means chosen to carry out the promise. The means are indirect only. The "Living Will" is one directive that many persons have drawn up to specify their wishes about treatment in the event they become comatose or otherwise unable to make directives or choices about treatment. Many Catholics have used the "Christian Affirmation of Life" to express their "desire not to have their lives prolonged by extraordinary medical procedures when they are terminally ill." It is not a legal document but is intended for devotional purposes. One paragraph says:

> I believe that God our Father has entrusted to me a shared dominion with him over my earthly existence so that I am bound to use ordinary means to preserve my life but I am free to refuse extraordinary means to prolong my life.

At stake are procedures which may benefit the patient as over against those which are optional or hold little prospect of aiding the patient's recovery. Catholic moralists define ordinary means as those which offer reasonable hope and benefit and do not involve excessive pain or illness. Extraordinary means are those which do not promise reasonable benefit and involve excessive cost, pain, or other considera-

ble inconvenience. Harmon Smith indicates a more pragmatic distinction: "Ordinary means are established medical
and surgical procedures appropriate to a given illness within
the limits of availability; extraordinary means are those
procedures (including medicines) which are incompletely established, frankly experimental, or bizarre."[23]

Since (1) the decision about the use of procedures belongs
finally to the doctors, (2) and since the Living Will statement
has legal standing in only a few states and even in those states
simply relieves physicians of legal vulnerability, and (3) since
the distinction between ordinary and extraordinary is so
vague, the statement has very little value in freeing the patient from extensive manipulation and repeated resuscitations.[24] Karen Ann Quinlan would not have been affected by
this since she had no terminal illness and she had left no
statement of her wishes. Even so, at least in those cases
where death is imminent the patient's wish not to be artificially sustained is to be respected. It does have the moral
force of declaring the patient's attitudes toward being artifically sustained. The moral claim should be respected, since
there is no moral tradition that says the physician is duty-
bound to prolong life.[25] The more widespread the concern
about treatment in excess of need and the depersonalizing
effects of machines that can keep patients "alive" even beyond senescence, the more the need for clarity at law will
become apparent. At present one can only hope to be mercifully spared the prospect of prolonged death by those who
will not detach the machines.

5. The fifth type of elective death is *passive, involuntary,
and direct:*[26] simple mercy killing without the request of the
patient and using direct means. Included would be instances
such as shooting a person trapped in a fire, smothering or
tranquilizing a defective newborn rather than force it to
starve to death, or terminating a patient in the agonizing
stages of a terminal illness such as Tay-Sachs disease, leukemia, or Huntington's chorea.

A woman in Belgium gave birth to a child with no arms and

with a badly deformed face, a condition caused by taking thalidomide in early pregnancy. Believing the child should not have to face life under such circumstances, the mother put barbiturates in the infant's formula and killed it. The mother and her physician were indicted and tried for murder, but were acquitted.[27]

Actions of this type are considered homicide under the legal codes of almost every country. Uruguay, while calling it a crime, provides for the penalty to be set aside. Fletcher points out that eleven cases of mercy killing have reached the courts of the United States: one on a charge of voluntary manslaughter, with conviction and penalty of three to six years' imprisonment and a $500 fine; another for first degree murder, with conviction but a penalty of six years in prison with immediate parole; the remaining nine were declared innocent by reason of "temporary insanity" or no-proof judgments.[28]

Morally such actions are extremely problematic. Anyone who promises to make a "death decision" for another is accepting grave responsibility. Few situations lend themselves to such abuses as those which give moral permission to take the life of another. Motives are also involved that may make the difference between acts which are morally blameworthy and those which are blameless. The delicate balance between a judgment to preserve the severely handicapped and the decision to terminate since the prospects for a meaningful life are slim may be tipped by an awareness of bothersome and prolonged therapeutic care, the appeal of estate settlements, or the prospects of more attractive sexual opportunities.

Proponents, while admitting the difficulty, still point to the principle recognized in both ethics and law that "the abuse of a thing does not rule out its use." Under certain circumstances the act can only be considered merciful. Where it is combined with or prompted by a profound interest in the personal well-being and integrity of the patient there is some question as to whether it is morally blameworthy. Certainly it is not to be considered in the category of criminal acts or branded as murder, which is killing with "malice afore-thought."

6. The final type of elective death is *passive, involuntary, and indirect.* Traditionally referred to simply as negative euthanasia, these are procedures that "let the patient go" by withdrawing or withholding life-preserving treatments.[29] The attending medical personnel may turn off a respirator, stop giving intravenous injections, withdraw drugs, or cancel an operation. Another means used by physicians to permit death to come more quickly for the patient is that of not treating a secondary illness contracted in the terminal stage of an illness. Thus, should an elderly patient suffering from cancer contract pneumonia, the physician may leave the pneumonia untreated and thus shorten the patient's life.

The decision to withhold treatment is ostensibly based upon mercy for the patient. The conclusion has been reached that it is better for the patient to die from pneumonia than to suffer the final agonizing stages of cancer. The secondary or complicating illness intervenes to shorten the period of suffering.

BIBLICAL PERSPECTIVES ON ELECTIVE DEATH

The fact that matters concerning both personal and public well-being are at stake in the euthanasia debate makes it imperative that the moral issues be weighed carefully and placed in biblical perspective. The literature on the subject shows that (1) both sides use the teaching of Scripture to provide warrants or justifications for their moral posture, and (2) there is no single or uniform answer among Christians that resolves the complex questions regarding elective death. What is at stake is not the sincerity with which one takes Scripture but competing visions of reality which both inform and are shaped by one's reading of Scripture. Personal experiences, perceptions of the situation, and theological perspectives all provide important filters for one's reading of the Bible.

The debate also largely centers on only certain types of elective death. General agreement can be found among even the most ardent opponents of euthanasia that (1) people have a moral right to refuse treatment, especially in those cases in which the illness is not curable; (2) it is right to withdraw, upon patient request, treatment that uses extraordinary means; and (3) it is morally justifiable to "let the patient go" and not strive to maintain vital signs after a patient is recognizably dead or dying. Thus, types 1, 4, and 6 are not critically at issue. In each of these cases, the patient dies as a result of disease and not as a direct result of action intended to kill or hasten dying.

This is the crucial distinction at stake in types 2, 3, and 5: the suicide, or self-killing; aiding another person's suicide or killing the person upon request; and directly killing a person without the person's request. These actions move beyond passive actions that "permit" dying to a direct action that knowingly and intentionally hastens or brings about death.

Some clarity might be brought to the debate by examining some of the variables that are involved in the arguments and their relationship to the biblical witness. There are at least three interrelated concerns: definition of personhood and "life"; attitudes toward death and divine providence; and the moral distinction between killing and allowing to die. Arguments pro and con involve theological or ground-of-meaning concerns and moral principles or rules. Perspectives on these issues will determine the moral position taken on the central question in the euthanasia debate, namely, whether death is, at least to some degree, elective.

Personhood and the Meaning of Life

The question of anthropology is at the heart of the euthanasia debate. Those who oppose any form of elective death argue that every life has some value and this is to be respected and protected as an unrepeatable gift. Each person is unique, and that life, once lost to death, cannot be replaced. This is the "sanctity of life" argument that holds life to be a gift from God to be held in trust. As God gives life, so he decides the time and circumstances of death. People do not have dominion over life or death. Such ultimate issues belong only to God.

Supporters of at least some forms of elective death begin with the notion that a fundamental element in what it means to be human is the ability to set the terms with death. While the "sanctity of life" argument defines dignity as the inviolability of life as vitality, the focus here is on human dignity as freedom, especially the freedom to interact with the events impinging upon one's life.

The Bible and Personhood. A theology of personhood is important in two ways: first, as a person confronting the reality and meaning of death, and, secondly, as a patient who is dying. The former deals with the person as a reflective moral agent, while the latter deals with the presence or absence of life that can meaningfully be called person. Whether and to what degree death can be considered elective raises the issue of whether such a decision belongs to what it means to be human.

The main features of the biblical portrait of person can be summarized briefly. First, the person is regarded as animated flesh—a living soul (Gen. 2:7). This underscores the importance of biology and animation to personhood. Second, people bear the image of God (Gen. 1:26–28) which distinguishes humankind from the rest of creation. People have godlike abilities or capacities which are not shared to the same degree by other creatures. These powers enable them to relate to God and fellow creatures and to understand—at least to a considerable degree—the processes of nature and history of which they are a part. People reflect upon their past history, their present circumstances, and their future prospects and relate personally to the activity of God in their lives.

The third feature of personhood is choice-making based upon moral reasoning (Gen. 3:22). Perceptions of right and wrong or good and evil must be considered before one engages in any act that would affect one's own self, the well-being of others, or the natural environment in which one lives.

Being created in the image of God, therefore, means to be fashioned with a "life" that has powers like those of God himself. This is the uniqueness of being human, and on this biblical portrait all Christian understandings of human dignity must be based. The person is one who is (1) alive, (2) related to others, (3) reflective, (4) able to make moral decisions, and (5) spiritual.[30] All these qualities are bound up in the notion of *imago Dei.*

However, some contenders in the euthanasia debate seem to reduce the notion of personhood to animation or to a biological form. Francis Schaeffer and C. Everett Koop never explicitly define what they mean by the term but apply it to include every instance of human life, including the comatose and brain dead.[31] This leads to the conclusion that one may never act to terminate "life," since that is "to destroy an *ikon* of God."[32]

This notion of *imago Dei* seems to be construed as an objective possession. It is the equivalent of the genetic argument in the abortion debate. The image is an entity given at conception and not lost until the heart and respiration cease, which is problematic on both logical and biblical grounds.

The equating of animation with the image of God has no biblical support. According to the creation narrative, the person as male and female was created "a living soul" (*nephesh chayyah,* Gen. 2:7). This term is also used to refer to animals, fish, and birds (1:20, 21, 24, where it is translated "living creatures"). If animation is *imago Dei,* all animal life would be the *ikons* of God.[33]

Furthermore, defining personhood in terms of breath or "life" could as logically be done with the notion of "blood." The relationship of breath to life is similar to the relationship between blood and life. Obviously one cannot be a person without either. However, neither can a person be reduced to either blood or breath. Biblical writers understood that "the blood is the life" (Deut. 12:23) and that "the life of every creature is the blood of it" (Lev. 17:14). They had observed that sacrificial animals and people died when blood was drained from their bodies. Thus, the blood flowing from the body was regarded as the flowing of life from the body. This important observation can hardly be denied. Some primitives made the reductionistic mistake, however, of reasoning that all of life's characteristics are therefore contained in the blood. Thus, Pliny recommended that epileptics drink the fresh, warm blood of a mortally wounded gladiator.

This was no less contrary to the biblical notion of life than are current efforts to define personhood by single biological criteria such as genetic code, breath, or heartbeat. The life of the person should be considered as a whole and not reduced to the lowest common biological denominator.[34] The larger problem, however, is that the complexity of the biblical portrait is reduced to a single feature. The Bible views personhood in a wholistic sense.

The person is a complex creature that defies simplistic definitions. Biology, mind, and spirit are inextricably related in ways that defy explanation but that result in a many-sided and wondrous creature with enormous powers of insight, hindsight, and foresight—abilities possessed by no other creature.

Death and Human Dignity. The capabilities of personhood take on special meaning where the reality of death is concerned. The dignity or grandeur of being a person involves relating to death in several ways. The phrase "death with dignity" reflects these concerns. At least three elements are involved. First, human dignity is at stake in being able to anticipate the coming of death. The question is not whether but when one is to die. That awareness is unique among people. All animals die, but only people live with the anxiety of that awareness. As Ramsey says, "The grandeur and misery of man are fused together in the human reality and experience of death."[35]

Secondly, dignity is basic to being able to prepare for death. "Set your house in order; for you shall die" (Isa. 38:1) is a universal moral and spiritual imperative. This involves spiritual preparation through repentance and faith, and practical preparation such as estate planning, the making of wills, and providing access to information for survivors. At this level, dignity involves making decisions about death based upon one's anticipations and calculations of the possibilities.

The Living Will was developed by and for people determined to anticipate and make some decision about the circumstances under which they might die. Those who sign such documents are exercising the distinctive human capacity of anticipating the fact that they might be kept alive far past the point of sentient existence. Their wish is to "be allowed to die and not kept alive by artificial means or heroic measures." This is based on the stated beliefs that (1) death is a part of reality, and (2) "the indignity of deterioration, dependence and hopeless pain" is a worse prospect than death itself.

Wayne Morse and Charles Lindbergh chose to die without elaborate medical procedures. The Van Dusens went even farther. Anticipating the loss of their mental faculties and refusing to become totally dependent upon others, they chose to set the terms with death and thus committed suicide.

Advocates of elective death argue that people, in making such decisions, are acting out the burden and responsibility of human dignity. Karen Ann Quinlan is unable to choose and thus is suffering the indignity of loss of personhood in her dying.

A third dimension of dignity involves accepting death with equanimity. This requires spiritual preparation, to be sure, but the aim is to accept the imminence of death without dread or terror. Saying that "death is nothing but dreadful to any human being"[36] is to reveal a very limited base of information. Studies of patients who have had positive life-after-life experiences show that their fear and dread of death practically disappeared. Elisabeth Kübler-Ross delayed publishing her findings precisely because she feared they would make death appear too attractive.

Some opponents of elective death argue that the very notion of death with dignity will erode the tenacity with which people cling to life and the determination of science to postpone death as long as possible. As Ramsey says, "The more acceptable in itself death is, the less the worth or uniqueness ascribed to the dying life."[37]

Surely, however, the consequences of accepting death with equanimity would far outweigh whatever disadvantages might accrue. The Bible makes it clear that fearing death can be a terrible and persistent bondage. The writer of Hebrews interpreted Jesus' death as destroying the evil power of the dread of death. Just as Jesus could face death victoriously, so could all those who faithfully follow the will of the Father (Heb. 2:14–15).

A person's moral resolve as well as human dignity is destroyed by anxiety about staying alive. Death's greatest victory is to reduce persons to whimpering victims of this universal sentence. Even the Son of God suffered the final indignity. But he did so with dignity. Confronting it squarely in the face, he refused to be intimidated by it.

People like the Van Dusens were acting on their beliefs concerning what it means to be a person making decisions before God about when it is appropriate to live and when it is appropriate to die. Their decision is a reminder that there are some ways of dying that enhance and affirm life and that more adequately symbolize the person's attitudes toward life, death, and the afterlife. Their note explaining the reasons for the decision ended with a prayer that set the action in the context of religious faith:

O Lamb of God, that takest away the sins of the world,
   have mercy on us;
O Lamb of God, that takest away the sins of the world,
   grant us thy peace.[38]

The Death of the Person. The second way in which the
question of personhood is raised concerns the patient who is
dying. Is there a point in the degenerative process toward
death beyond which one ceases to be a truly human person?
Just as it is difficult to recognize the earliest stages of fetal life
as "person," so it is difficult to define as "person" one whose
body is being totally supported by mechanical/chemical
means. James B. Nelson has helpfully distinguished three
stages on the continuum between conception and death. The
pre-personal denotes the early stage of gestation, prior to the
development of sufficient biological capacities for the fetus to
be regarded as person. The personal is that stage of human
life during which an individual is cognitive, functioning, and
interactive with others. The post-personal is that stage during which the dying patient "has irretrievably lost its capacity for personhood."[39]

The question is important for determining the extent of
moral obligation to sustain medically a patient who is dying.
The problem is posed because science now has the ability to
maintain the vital life signs of heartbeat and respiration long
after the brain has ceased to function. One man was resuscitated twice while on a ventilator even after the neurosur-
geon had refused to examine the patient because the brain
was dead. Those who insist on such heroic measures are
focusing only on "life signs" and not on the "person." These
actions force patients into a vegetative state. Advocates of
elective death argue that preserving life regardless of circumstances is to love an abstraction ("life") rather than a
person. Care for the person requires concern for personality
as well as vital life signs. To do less is to slip inevitably into
a biological idolatry.

The problem remains, however, as to *when* that line is crossed between personal human life and human life. Morally, the distinction is critical. As Ramsey says, the real question in euthanasia is, "When in the continuum of the dying process there is still life among us who lays claim to the immunities, respect and protection which in ethics and/or by law are accorded by man to fellow man?"[40] There is more agreement on the question than on its answer. The issue concerns the "life" that "lays claim" upon us. Elsewhere, Ramsey acknowledges that the mere presence of life signs does not lay the claim of "necessity to preserve" upon physicians. Speaking of whether to use extraordinary measures to preserve defective neonates, he suggests that the principle that should be posed is:

> Whether it is not morally responsible, or at least morally tolerable, to negate some of the negative consequences of the practice of saving life. Should not the practice be limited by the sort of respect that esteems life enough to allow it to die on occasion even if it technically could be saved?[41]

Thus, not every instance of life should be kept alive, and not everything that could be done should be done. The moral responsibility toward the patient varies with the stage in the dying process and the patient's wishes with regard to treatment based upon personal, moral, and religious beliefs.

Dying is a process rather than an event.[42] In one sense, the degenerative process is going on all the time, of course. Some have used this as a flip argument that "since we are all dying, why not terminate anyone?" This is sophistry; a clever but nonserious attempt to avoid the issue. The question concerns those who are facing imminent death.

There are several dimensions or stages to this process. *Clinical death* takes place when respiration and heartbeat cease. Resuscitation may restore meaningful life to the patient at this stage, as numerous, happy cases have shown. Such restorations have enabled studies to be made of patient experiences "while dead." Tragically, however, clinical reversal has also led to the restoring of vital signs when the brain has been so damaged that no possibility of conscious personal existence remains, as in the Quinlan case. *Brain death* begins to occur soon after cardiac failure or may happen from other injury apart from cardiopulmonary arrest. The first functions to die are those which control consciousness, followed by those which control the nervous system and heart-lung functions. *Biological death* is the stage of permanent loss of the body's ability to sustain cardiac and respiratory function. Even so, some cellular structures such as hair and fingernails will continue to grow, so it is necessary to speak of *cellular death,* as the final stage.[43]

When in this process does one cross the line between personal human life and human life? Little, if any, specific guidance is provided by the Bible on this question. We are dealing with a dilemma never confronted by the biblical writers—the ability to prolong life far beyond the point at which death would normally or naturally have occurred. The new technology of medicine is able to do with medical apparatus what our biblical forebears had to do on their own, namely, breathe. Should the normative clue be taken from the fact that people in biblical times were declared dead when their breathing stopped, many of the "advances" in medicine would either never have been possible, should never have been used, or should immediately be destroyed. Few people believe that should be done, however, grateful as we are that science has been able to restore healthy life to persons who had died from acute illness or were suffering from chronic disease. Reversing clinical death (heart arrest) has often given many additional years of meaningful living to people who would have irretrievably died in biblical times.

What is required is that imagination, intuition, and reflection bridge the time-and-circumstance distance between the biblical writers and those now confronting the dilemma of dying. The contemporary disciple is required to render a response that captures the essence of faith without a slavish or neurotic need to have the Bible provide the answer. Indeed, it cannot. There are no specific parallels in the Bible, nor is there an attempt to give definitive answers to the specific dilemmas of our time. The Bible provides guidance and guidelines; it is not a lexicon of specific decisions required of the faithful.

The crucial dilemma arises in those difficult cases where science is still helpless to offer any prospect for recovery or restoration of health. For all its benefits, science has not and will not abolish death. But it can delay the time when death is obvious. The machine has extended the zone between life and death and made it difficult to determine when a patient should be declared dead.

The biblical concern for the person as a psychosomatic whole seems to require that human death be comprehended personally and interpersonally as well as bodily-biologically.[44] Biological activity may be basic to but is not the same as personal human life. Personhood is more than the vital signs. Callahan states it strongly:

> Genetically, a body still circulating blood is in some sense a "human life," if genetic membership in the human species is the norm. Then, if the moral aim is to preserve whatever genetically counts as "individual human life," then an artificially sustained body meets the standard. But if the moral concern is with personhood—thus presupposing our electrically active brain—then, in the absence of brain activity, no "person" is present.[45]

Christians will give moral support to those medical procedures which hold some promise of preserving personal human life. However, there is no biblical basis for insisting that patients be sustained as long as there are vital signs. The current equivalent of the biblical criteria for death in the absence of breath or the loss of blood (Lev. 17:14; Deut. 12:23) may well be in brain death. All the features associated with the biblical portrait of person rest in the higher functions of the brain. This includes "potentiality for significant personal life, for some relationship to God, and for interrelationships with other human beings."[46]

By this standard, support can be given the recommendation by the President's Commission for the Study of Ethical Problems in Medicine and Biomedical and Behavioral Research for Congress and the states to adopt "brain death" statutes. This would be in addition to or instead of the traditional statute based on heart stoppage. Already twenty-seven states have done so.[47] This would have avoided the agony of the parents of Andra Rubinelli, who went to court to have her declared legally dead. She was being maintained on a respirator even though her brain was dead. While the judge deliberated the case for two weeks, Andra's heart stopped, thus resolving the question.[48] Indiana law recognizes only heart death. The parents were concerned about Andra as a person. The dilemma could be avoided in such cases by the adoption of a wholistic understanding of personhood and death rather than insisting upon a vitalistic definition of life.

Personhood and the Meaning of Death

The second major area of concern in the debate over elective death relates to personhood and the meaning of death. This involves a cluster of problems including theological perspectives about death, the special dimensions of death for people, and whether God alone controls the moment of death. The place to begin is to recognize that moral responsibility is directly linked to human capacities of reflective choice. Where there is no choice, there is no responsibility to choose. But the higher degree or level of responsiveness, the higher degree or level of responsibility for choices that reflect moral or spiritual commitments.

The responsibility for making decisions regarding death and dying belongs to the unique ability among human beings to come to terms with the reality of death. While all living things die, death has special meaning to people. Only people know that they are to die. Death is the constant companion of mortality and people must live with that awareness. This special knowledge of death in the human future adds a special burden to being human.

This also involves the moral dimensions of elective death —those instances in which people act as instruments or agents to cause death. The biblical story of the first murder (Gen. 4:8) was, of course, not the first instance of killing among God's creatures. It is the first conscious reflection upon the morality of taking another person's life. This creature made in the image of God is portrayed as self-consciously analyzing the religious or moral dimensions of killing. People make choices based upon moral reflection. They are not driven out of necessity or instinct alone but may understand the dynamics involved and choose accordingly. The consequences of these choices may also be calculated. When killing is motivated by selfishness, pride, anger, or greed, it is sinful, results in guilt and alienation from God, and entails judgment.

Furthermore, a fear of dying may pervade human consciousness and lead to despair. This "worm at the core of human existence" (William James) may appear a cruel joke played on the knower by the Creator. Camus concluded that such a knowledge without the certainty of survival beyond death leads inevitably and logically to the conclusion that life is meaningless—absurd. Such despair is ultimate sin, for it denies the hope at the core of the biblical faith. As the apostle Paul expressed it: "If for this life only we have hoped in Christ, we are of all men most to be pitied" (I Cor. 15:19).

The biblical answer to the special problem posed by death is the hope of resurrection. To be sure, one mystery is juxtaposed against another. The questions posed by one reality are answered by the greater mystery surrounding the truth of resurrection. Death is neither more real nor more ultimate, however, simply because its experience is universally painful. The cross of Good Friday may loom larger and darker because of its pathos and tragedy, but it gains its larger meaning only by the deeper mystery of the resurrection hope.

Death must be taken with radical seriousness but not given ultimate standing. The biblical faith is a resurrection faith, placing death in the larger scheme of life. This is why death cannot be held to be an ultimate threat to well-being. Ramsey's reflection on the death of Stewart Alsop captured the pathos of human anxiety and loss but ended in despair. "Death," he said, "[is] an irreparable loss, an unquenchable grief, the threat of all threats, a dread that is more than all fears aggregated together, an approaching 'evil' which annuls every ordinary distinction between good and evil."[49]

Death: The Last Enemy? Such annihilism is nonbiblical because it holds no hope perspective that transcends and thus transforms the threat of death. Death can be "an irreparable loss" only if it is thought of as an ultimate enemy and always an evil.

The apostle Paul's statement that "the last enemy to be destroyed is death" (I Cor. 15:26) is frequently cited to support this view. This is linked with the argument that death entered the world as a punishment for sin.[50] Proof for this is also found in Paul where he says that "the wages of sin is death" (Rom. 6:23).

Following this clue, some scientists have resolved to eradicate death from the human experience.[51] They rightly perceive that science has a moral mandate to try to eradicate death if it is an ultimate enemy. The biblical promise of eternal life (i.e., immortality) awaits the dawn of the technological wizardry that would usher in the age in which death would be no more (see Rev. 21:4). The eschatological kingdom envisioned by the writers of the New Testament becomes the goal and purpose for the world of science. The aim is to remove death as a sentence passed upon everyone and make it an option which only an unhappy minority would elect.

Such efforts seem more a sign of anxiety in the face of death[52] than the result of moral sensitivity to the will of God. At most, the Bible gives warrants for extending or prolonging life that is meaningful. Death not only cannot but should not be eliminated from human experience. It cannot, for it belongs to finitude and mortality. It should not, for death is as necessary to the processes of nature and the ongoing of history as is birth.

This argument is also based upon a misreading of Scripture. Paul's statement about death is that it is the *last* enemy to be defeated. "Last" is *eschatos,* meaning the last in a series (see Matt. 12:45; also Luke 11:26 and II Peter 2:20). There is no hint that death is an *ultimate* enemy.

Notice also that Paul is not arguing that (biological) death is the consequence of sin. In his writings (and elsewhere), death is used in two ways. One is biological. Death means the cessation of animation. The second is what might best be termed "spiritual." Death here means the absence of the true life—the life eternal which is the gift of God. This John spoke of as *zoe* (see I John 3:11–18). The absence of this quality extended into eternity is eternal death. These meanings are often used to play on the meaning of "life." Those who do not have the life of God are spoken of as "dead"— even though they are obviously animated, having breath and heartbeat.

In reading biblical texts, one must be aware of this variety of meanings, the interplay between them, and the interaction of the terms "death" and "life" with their nuances. Failure to do so accounts in part for the notion that Paul held that death in the biological sense was the consequence of sin (Rom. 3:23; 5:21). The parallelism Paul is employing, however, makes it clear that he is speaking of spiritual death as the consequence of sin: "For the wages of sin is death, but the free gift of God is eternal life in Christ Jesus our Lord" (Rom. 6:23). Elsewhere he speaks of those who are living apart from Christ as "dead in trespasses and sins" (Eph. 2:1). The corollary is his speech about "eternal life as the gift of God's grace." Just as "life" is not animation, neither is death biological. Both death and life are moral concepts or references to spiritual realities.

Death as the loss of animation is the consequence of creation and mortality. The creation narratives clearly state that Adam and Eve were expelled from the garden *before* they ate the fruit of the tree of life which would make them live forever (Gen. 3:22). To be created is to be mortal and to be mortal is to have finite limits. Even if Adam and Eve had not sinned, they would have come to an end. Death belongs to creation. The Genesis account assumes the mortality of man and does not include death as a consequence of sin. God's address to Adam that "you are dust, and to dust you shall return" (Gen. 3:19b) was a reminder of his origins and not a new factor created by his sin.[53] Even Paul's account of cosmic redemption does not relate the termination of physical existence on earth to sin (Rom. 8:18–25).[54]

To argue that death is the consequence of sin implies that creation is evil. Consistent with the Hebrew notion of the goodness of creation, Paul never says the body is evil, however. Finitude may be a source of human anxiety, but it is not the cause of sin.

The dualism of the Scriptures is not cosmic but moral. Death is not the creation of an evil power nor even of the sinful rebellion of man the creature. Death is a part of creation, howbeit a painful part. The pain of death stems from two sources. One is the loss of relationship created by the death of loved ones. The pain is in the survivor, however, not in the deceased. Again the pain of death is related to what it means to be human. The loss of every person is felt in the depths of human community. Presumably this level of pain is not felt by most of earth's creatures. Certainly it is not experienced to the same degree, for only human beings can ponder its meaning and contemplate its approach. Those dimensions are uniquely human.

The second source of the pain of death is sin. Human sin pervades and corrupts all relationships. Certainly at times death is the direct result of sin, as in war, homicide, reckless driving, a poisoned environment, etc. More often it is an indirect cause—human sinfulness in rebellion against the finality of death. Resistance to death in the sense of denying its reality is itself sinful, for that is rebellion against the bounds of creaturely finitude. To seek to be as the gods, i.e., immortal, is to strive after that which the creature is not. Sin is also present in the death-denying strategies invented by modern minds and always lurking just beneath the surface of the human consciousness. Refusing to accept the fact that our history is bracketed by birth and death is sinful. This rebellion is at the root of many of the desperate medical ministrations employed when a patient dies or wants to die. Striving "officiously to keep alive" may be a sign of the denial of death and a refusal to accept the limitations of human dominion over every facet of existence in creation.

Such tragic desperation may be cleverly disguised as concern for the patient. However, when the patient has expressed the desire that no extraordinary measures be used, it cannot be that such procedures are responsive to covenantal agreements between doctor and patient. The contrary is true: covenant is violated and trust has been betrayed. In such cases, doctors are dealing with their own fears—not with the needs of the patient.[55]

The problem is illustrated by the story of a sixty-eight-year-old doctor who was dying of an inoperable cancer of the stomach. The patient developed a pulmonary embolism, which was then surgically removed. After collapsing from a myocardial infarction, the patient was revived by a cardiac resuscitation team. This happened four times in succession. Then, for several weeks the patient was maintained in spite of severe brain damage following the cardiac arrests and episodes of vomiting accompanied by generalized convulsions.

The doctor-patient knew he had stomach cancer, which he accepted with equanimity though he was in severe pain because the cancer had spread to the bone. He responded with gratitude at the removal of the embolism but asked that no further attempts be made to resuscitate him should he expire. His request was (obviously) denied.[56] The sin in this case is twofold: first, in that the man's request was disregarded, which is a breach of trust in doctor-patient relations, and second, in that too much was done in resisting the coming of death.

This man was denied his wish to die even though he fully understood the nature of his illness and the inevitable outcome. No artificial or clever arguments of moral principles and medical ethics can camouflage the evil of subjecting this patient to the indignity of artificial medical ministrations that were dehumanizing and depersonalizing. Sin may be in doing too much, as it is in doing too little.

Leave Death to God? To insist on human passivity in the face of death seems a denial of God's work and purpose in creation and redemption. The one thing for which God has clearly worked through millennia is to fashion a creature that will not be simply the passive victim of fate or circumstance. To argue that "death should be left in the hands of God" seems a pious dodge to avoid the responsible decision-making that the imminence of death requires.

Notice the problems. First, the argument is inconsistent, since medical science is encouraged to do all in its power to keep the patient alive. If, in fact, the death decision is God's alone, the medical apparatus would have to be withdrawn entirely. Such intervention seems at times "to 'war without retreat and without quarter' against almighty God for the last shred of sentient life."[57] Since death would come more quickly and "naturally" as a result of debilitated physiological processes and since God's will regarding a particular death is considered the cessation of those processes, the matter is certainly not simply "up to God." All medical science is a matter of playing God, which means making life-and-death decisions and taking responsibility for them.

A second problem is that God's action in creating choice makers is being denied. The assumption is that persons can only choose to maintain "life" but never choose "death." This is to counsel a fatalism that makes people victims of chance and circumstances rather than creatures who are required to have dominion over nature and its course. The knowledge that people have regarding the causes and processes of death and their ability to calculate the course of the dying process give a special responsibility for acting on the basis of that knowledge. The ethical question is whether we can justify a fatalistic and passive posture toward whatever happens to us.

The Christian notion of stewardship holds that people are called to a working relationship—a co-partnership—with God. The processes of nature are to be understood as perfectly as possible *for the purpose* of exercising dominion or diminishing the evil effects of what those processes might do to people. People are to discern the circumstances when it is imperative to choose life and when it is futile (and perhaps immoral) to strive against the inevitability of death. God works through people to accomplish his loving purposes. Whether we choose to continue treatment or to refrain from it; whether to allow to die or to actively aid the person's dying, the choice should be in response to God's care.

A third problem relates to the nature of God. Human suffering poses the dilemma of divine providence, especially as it pertains to excessive or dysfunctional pain. The assertion that God has caused certain people to die an agonizing death is difficult, if not impossible, to square with the biblical understanding that "God is love" (I John 4:8).

Certainly, in the Christian perspective, suffering may serve the purpose of God. Job was brought to a new and more profound level of humility and worship (Job 42:1–6), and Jesus himself was made perfect through suffering (Heb. 2:10). Death can be the final stages of growth, as Kübler-Ross has illustrated,[58] during which lessons can be learned and personal insight enhanced.

Speaking of this "pedagogy of death," some argue that the patient should not be robbed of the final stages of living (dying) lest the person lose the benefits that such suffering can bring.[59] Reflecting on Alsop's coming to terms with "Uncle Thanatos,"[60] Ramsey says that he "gained both in solidarity with humankind and in appreciation for the uniqueness of his own and others' individual existence."[61] Norman St. John-Stevas believes the incurably ill should be sustained—even in their pain—to learn lessons otherwise to be missed. "The final stages of an incurable illness can be a vast wasteland," he wrote, "but it need not be. It can be a vital period in one's life reconciling him to life and to death and giving him an interior peace."[62]

There are important moral and theological differences between acknowledging that growth *may* take place through the dying process and insisting that persons *must* suffer even unrelievable pain because they need to grow! This argument has several obvious flaws in logic. First, many patients no longer have the capacity for learning, since their brain is already dead. Second, little, if any, learning can take place when pain is excruciating and unrelievable, as in cases of cancer of the throat. Pain does not always result in stronger faith but may drive the person to despair and disbelief. Suffering may be totally dysfunctional. Finally, lessons may have been learned already by the person facing death. Insisting that their suffering be prolonged is to stand between the dying and their relationship to God—a type of religious imperialism.

The question of God's intention for spiritual growth on the part of his children should be separated from the question of whether God wills or causes extensive pain and suffering. We can say with certainty that God wills the good of all who suffer (Rom. 8:28). But we are less certain as to precisely how God is working in the midst of unrelievable pain. We can be sure, however, that God is not the *cause* of every human tragedy. The Book of Job insisted that God did not cause Job to suffer. That was the action of "the adversary," Satan (Job 2:7). It cannot be argued that God causes all painful dying. That would be to say immoral things about God, who knows how to give good things to his children (Matt. 7:11). As Eike-Henner W. Kluge says, "It is simply incredible to consider agony and undignified, even mindless suffering a deliberate means whereby an omniscient, omnipotent and omnibenevolent deity wishes to develop virtue in either sufferer or onlooker."[63]

Far from willing or causing tragic suffering, God provides death as a way of escape in the event one's life becomes unbearably tragic. Five men in the Old Testament chose death by suicide rather than face the extended and non-redemptive sufferings of torture, humiliation, and public execution. Samson (Judg. 16:28–30), Saul (I Sam. 31:4–5), and others (see II Sam. 17:23; I Kings 16:8–18) chose a quick death rather than slow death. Not one of these stories suggests that suicide was unforgivable. The persons decided on the basis of their religious faith and their belief concerning the appropriate time to die.

Death can be a good gift. Job gained strength to endure his pain in part by the awareness that he could choose death (Job 3:13). Paul also seemed to suggest that death had a positive side. He spoke of the sting of death (I Cor. 15:56), but also saw it as a way to escape his tribulation and be with the Father (Phil. 1:23). He actually indicated he preferred death to the suffering he was undergoing, saying that it was only for the sake of those to whom he ministered that he would remain alive. Although the text is unclear, he seemed to intimate that the choice was his to make (Phil. 1:22).

As a gift of the sovereign grace of God, death has a redemptive and redeeming side. God's good purposes may be served through death, and his mercy may be experienced as the blessed release from unnecessary suffering. This is why a friend at a church in Kentucky expressed her profound gratitude to God for having relieved her husband from the excruciating pain of terminal cancer. Far from being a dread to every person, death may be welcomed or invited as a friend, a welcome gift from God.

Killing vs. Allowing to Die

The third major area of debate concerns the moral distinction between killing and allowing to die. On this question, the debate operates at the rules level, frequently appealing to the biblical commandment "You shall not kill" (Ex. 20:13). Those who see this commandment as a rule permitting no exception in medical practice argue that there is an absolute moral distinction between killing and allowing the patient to die. Those who advocate some form of active euthanasia see the commandment as a summary rule that provides general guidance but not an absolute rule for every case. The commandment establishes an important presumption against killing.[64] It recognizes that most cases of killing are morally unjustifiable or reprehensible, as in mass murder. Even so, that does not mean that killing is always wrong. It may at times be justifiable as the lesser of two evils or the right and morally required act.

In both cases, the rule about killing is dialectically related to theological convictions and assumptions about the meaning of life and death. Thus the debate also involves theological or ground-of-meaning assumptions.

The Biblical Commandment. The biblical injunction not to kill establishes a moral constraint on human freedom by limiting the types of actions that are permitted toward fellow human beings. This is a necessary constraint to remind society of the moral and legal protection required for those who are vulnerable from age, disease, injury, or incapacitating illness. William E. May extends this to argue that euthanasia would destroy community, since it would undermine the trust between people that is necessary for covenant concern and protection.[65]

Several problems emerge, however, when one examines the biblical commandment itself as used in the euthanasia debate. First, the commandment does not proscribe all killing. The same law that forbids killing also allows capital punishment for nine different crimes (Ex. 21:12–17, 29; Lev. 20:2–16), killing in wars that are either defensive or offensive in nature (Deuteronomy 20; I Samuel 15), and for killing in self-defense (Ex. 22:2). Thus, the commandment cannot be made an absolute rule on biblical grounds alone.

Secondly, the commandment is designed to protect those

who are not dying. It was designed to prohibit murder or the killing of another individual by a person who had no authorization from the community for doing so. John Yoder argues that it prohibited the death penalty as executed according to tribal codes. The proper authority or basis of decision-making in matters of life and death was not the individual or the clan, but the covenant community.[66] Thus, the commandment itself does not deal with the morality of mercy in aiding the dying. This poses a special problem for those who wish to use this text either to justify or condemn mercy killing. Certainly it cannot be used to "settle the question" as if all that were needed is obedience to the biblical commandment.

"Do no harm." Recognizing the problems inherent in applying the commandment, writers like Paul Ramsey and Arthur Dyck move to the "do no harm" principle of medical ethics.[67] A vow still taken by many physicians states: "I will use treatment to help the sick according to my ability and judgment, but never with a view to injury and wrongdoing. Neither will I administer a poison to anybody when asked to do so, nor will I suggest such a course."

Several problems are obvious in using this oath for contemporary Christian morality. The first is the problem of substituting the ethics of Hippocrates for the ethics of Jesus. "Do no harm" is a philosophical, not a biblical, principle. While this may be a valid moral principle, precisely how that becomes normative for Christian ethics needs more explanation. At a minimum, it is necessary to show how this rule is an extension of or is consistent with the norm of *agape,* Christlike love. Another problem is the selectivity used in isolating only this rule from the oath. It also prohibits surgery for kidney stones and giving any medical training to any person except "my sons, and the sons of my teacher and to pupils who have signed the indenture and sworn obedience to the 'physician's laws.' "[68]

Of greater importance is the intention and meaning of the oath. It does not deal with killing out of mercy; it forbids killing with malice. The fact that physicians might be tempted to use their skills to injure the unsuspecting and vulnerable patient is recognized. The physician swore not to aid the suicidal, nor to conspire with a third party to dispatch a patient. Medicine should not become a partner to crime, and physicians should not barter their expertise in training to those who would like to camouflage the crime of murder.

Finally, the Christian moral principle of neighbor love is a positive rule, not a negative one. It is a matter of doing good (Matt. 5:44; Acts 10:38; Rom. 7:13; Gal. 6:10), not just refraining from doing "harm." Furthermore, the good act is the requirement of mercy (Prov. 11:17; Luke 6:36; 10:37). This positive perspective permeates the pronouncements of Jesus. The Golden Rule is a summary statement of what is required: "Whatever you wish that men would do to you, do so to them" (Matt. 7:12; Luke 6:31). Certainly the prohibitive posture has a valuable emphasis. There are evils to be avoided. The positive requirement is both more demanding and more exacting, however. "Doing good" can never be reduced to "do no harm." The good act is required; it is not simply a matter of refusing to do what one perceives as forbidden.

The Golden Rule seems to teach that the measure of the act that is required is the action one would desire for oneself. Plainly the standard is not in some objective rule prohibiting certain acts. The good action can only be calculated by the imagination prompted by love for neighbor. That love is an outgoing goodwill that seeks the well-being of the neighbor, or seeks to act in mercy to meet the need of the neighbor.

A Paradigm: The Good Samaritan. Defining precisely what is permitted and what actions are prohibited by the twin requirements of love and mercy is never easy. Jesus' story of the Samaritan (Luke 10:29–37) illustrates the requirement but leaves the limits open to the intuitive faith of the believer. Opponents in the euthanasia debate turn to this story to gain support.

Marvin Kohl argues that helping someone die may well be what mercy requires. For him, if the motive is love, and the method chosen is a painless aid to quick death to benefit the patient, it would be morally acceptable.[69] The only types of cases he includes are (1) those involving patients dying from an incurable illness involving extensive pain who have expressed their desire for an easy death, and (2) those infants born not dying nor in intense pain but severely handicapped and without a functioning cerebral cortex. He feels that accepting the responsibility for acting in such extreme cases belongs to the patient-physician covenant. Helping such patients die is an act of kindness; refusing to do so would be cruel and unkind. The good Samaritan is his paradigm: love for neighbor may include euthanasia.

Dyck argues that "doing no evil" (nonmaleficence) is a stronger part of the Samaritan story than is "doing good." He also (wrongly) construes the rule as "Do not do to others what you would not want them to do to you."[70] He says the story includes the principle of not killing, which he regards as part of the total effort to prevent the destruction of human beings and human communities.

Jesus' story was an expansion on the meaning of his teaching to "love . . . your neighbor as yourself" (Luke 10:27). Dyck is right in saying that there is "nothing in the story that suggests that killing is a form of mercy or kindness." There can be no question that the injured Jew required care in the story as Jesus told it. The point raised by Kohl, however, is whether killing might ever be used in the service of love and mercy.

Dyck denies that possibility and cannot bring himself to think the Samaritan might possibly have acted differently. He builds his case for benemortasia (good dying) on an absolute moral distinction between killing and allowing to die. All that one is permitted to do for a dying patient is to (1) relieve pain, (2) relieve suffering, (3) respect the person's right to refuse treatment, and (4) provide health care regardless of cost. These permit one to be as beneficent as possible without violating the principle of nonmaleficence, he argues.[71]

Paul Ramsey also insists on an absolute moral distinction

between killing and allowing to die. Never could he permit intervening to hasten the patient's death, though he does say the dying should not be extended by artificial or heroic means. Mercy requires "simply to comfort and company with them, to be present to them."[72] The term he coins for this ethic of "only caring for the dying" is agathanasia.

Both Kohl and Dyck have to push the story of the good Samaritan beyond its limits to argue their positions. But Kohl more accurately understands the dilemma created by the requirement for mercy than does Dyck. Certainly, the Samaritan had no warrant-requirement for killing the injured Jew. The "patient" was not terminal—thus he hardly fits the case that poses the problem. *That* patient required care that involved the use of whatever medical techniques were available then. But might a modern "Samaritan" not sense a further, more burdensome and tragic moral responsibility in an encounter with a "patient" who is dying and who under conditions of extreme pain requests aid in dying?

Might Mercy Require Killing? Two problems emerge from Dyck and Ramsey's treatment. First is the insistence that helping a person die is "doing harm," or maleficence. For their approaches, a ground-of-meaning association is employed which is never explored, namely, a particular theology of death. This has been explored above. Whether aiding a person to die is to do harm is a matter of judgment not as easily resolved as Dyck and Ramsey would have us believe. Is it more harm to kill a patient who is (1) dying, (2) has no chance of recovery, (3) is in unrelievable pain, and (4) has requested help in dying, or to force that person to go on suffering, helpless to do anything about it, and hopelessly frustrated at having earnest, sincere, and rational requests repeatedly denied? Are agathanasia and benemortasia merciful, or do they stop short of what mercy may truly require?

Saul, when he saw he was defeated, (1) knew he was going to die at the hand of the enemy and (2) requested that he be slain by his armor-bearer (I Sam. 31:1–6). No mention was made of mercy in his request. Presumably he preferred to

die at the hand of his friend and caring servant than to die
after the humiliation, torture, and prolonged suffering he
was certain to receive from the hated Philistines. The armor-
bearer refused, "for he feared greatly" (v. 4).[73] Apparently,
it was not a matter of doing wrong but of cowardice. The
"greater harm" for Saul was to fall into the hands of the
enemy, where he would receive neither respect nor mercy.
There are times when prolonging "life" may be nothing
more than extending the time of needless suffering.

The Bible also places a strong emphasis on motive in actions. The difference in whether an act is right or wrong may
be determined by the motive involved. Evil intentions or
selfish motives may make an otherwise acceptable action
wrong. Building upon this insight, James Rachels has argued
that there is no absolute moral distinction between killing
and allowing to die.[74] A man who stands to inherit a fortune
if a brother dies is morally guilty whether he kills him directly or, if seeing him knocked unconscious and fallen into
a pool of water, refuses to rescue him and thus lets him
drown. Similarly, Rachels says, a doctor who lets a patient die
for loving and merciful reasons is in the same moral position
as if he had given the patient a lethal injection of drugs as an
act of love and mercy.

It is important to notice that Rachels argues that, generally
speaking, killing is worse than letting die. There are times,
however, when killing may be less reprehensible than allowing to die. Thus the moral distinction between allowing and
helping a patient to die is not always relevant.

This can be seen, for instance, when physicians decide to
allow a patient to die by not treating a secondary illness. A
patient who is dying of cancer may well contract pneumonia
or the flu. The physician may decide *out of mercy* to allow
the pneumonia to go untreated and thus shorten the time
required to die. Since the physician made the death decision,
should he have put an end to the patient's suffering by the
use of pain-killing drugs?

The Roman Catholic principle of double effect recognizes

the role of mercy in aiding death in cases of an incurable, painful illness. As Pope Pius XII said:

> Morals evidently condemn mercy-killing, that is, the intention of causing death. But if a dying person consents, it is permissible to use, with moderation, narcotics that will allay his suffering, but will also cause quicker death. . . . In this case, death is not the direct intention.[75]

The rule is designed both to give moral permission to hasten death and to restrain the killing of patients even out of mercy. Certainly it provides a psychological buffer for those uneasy about actually aiding a person to die.

However, the fact (1) that the patient is dying and (2) that administering the drugs will almost certainly bring death are known to the attending physician. Here is obviously a formal construct designed to give permission for a morally required act, namely, relieving pain even if it means death. Honesty compels the recognition, however, that the direct-indirect distinction breaks down. This is an act of *deliberately* easing into death. It is euthanasia by another name.[76] Plainly it recognizes that the moral distinction between killing and allowing to die is not absolute.[77]

The Tragic Requirement of Love? Ramsey and Dyck also recognize that killing is sometimes morally justified. In war, for instance, the Christian may have to set aside the predisposition not to kill and be obedient to "the countervailing requirements of *agape.*"[78] This is true even though killing under any circumstances is a *prima facie* violation of agape.[79] Even so, responsibility for the neighbor requires being willing to kill those who threaten life.

Both writers argue that self-defense and resisting the harm intended by the enemy justify killing in war. The same line of reasoning could have led them to different conclusions regarding the morality of euthanasia. Might it not be argued that one's predisposition not to kill may be set aside at the request of a dying patient who now *needs* an action other than those types of acts which prolong suffering or delay death? If one can include killing as an act of love in self-defense and the defense of others, could killing not also be included as an act of love toward one who desires death under certain conditions? Certainly such an act is rooted in a good motive, and thus is not murder.

Furthermore, suggestions for guidelines to govern the decision to directly terminate a patient might be drawn from those which people like Ramsey and Dyck use to guide decisions about war. The "just war" theory holds that, before one may kill at war on moral grounds, the war must meet the basic criteria of justifiable *cause* and justifiable *conduct.*[80]

Such principles suggest guidelines that might be followed in deciding to actively terminate a patient. As to *cause,* the action must involve the twin elements of beneficent motive with no ill will toward the patient and the condition of the patient who is dying or whose life is unbearably tragic. The *conduct* required is the caring administration of painless death—no torture or pain-inducing agents would be permitted. The means should be aesthetically acceptable.[81] The principles could be expanded. *Proper authority* would require status in the health care team, such as that of the attending physician, and acting on the authority of the family or nearest relative. It would also include those "Samaritans" who enter that circle of moral responsibility by chance or circumstance. The action would be *a last resort* when there is no reasonable hope for patient recovery to personal existence. And, on balance, the goods achieved—the cessation of pain, the relief from suffering, and those factors which pertain to family well-being—will outweigh the "evils" that are inevitable, e.g., the loss of a loved one to death, the pain of grief, and the suffering of loneliness.

Needless to say, the use of such criteria in themselves becomes a burdensome and loathsome constraint to moral action if the criteria are applied legalistically and rigidly. But they have the value of pointing to certain recognizable, although general, circumstances under which the moral obligation in patient care may slip inevitably from "keep alive" to "help to die." That these criteria can never be perfectly applied or that they never assure a perfect obedience is as true in medicine as it is in the politics of war. But that there is the "other side" of patient care and the moral obligation to aid one's dying can hardly be denied. To reject that difficult and terrifying dimension of moral obligation is to retreat from the exacting and complex requirements of love in the exceptional case.

CONCLUSION

The revolution in science and medicine has brought about a new epoch in the person's relation to death. Plainly the traditional approaches to death which leave the matter to chance or circumstance or totally "in the hands of God" are being challenged as to their adequacy. Such an approach does not adequately account for human responsibility for decisions relating to death and dying. Further, traditional answers to the requirements of love and mercy concerning medical care for the ill may not lead only to the conclusion that death must be postponed.

The advocates of elective death argue cogently that the demands of love and care for the patient go beyond "keeping alive." The possibility of repeated resuscitations without the prospect of recovery present a specter more to be feared than death for many thoughtful persons. What needs to be discovered are the countervailing requirements of agape. As Nelson says:

> If we can contemplate the precarious possibility that in *some* cases killing may be an act of merciful love and an expression of God's humanizing intentions for life, then we are resting neither in a life worship which is blind to life's quality nor in a death fear which is blind to transcendent hope.[82]

Love certainly will continue to demand that persons be cared for and respected by the artful uses of the healing sciences. Intensive care units will continue to serve as signs that the human community cares for those who are infirm and helpless, whose worth rests not on functional value but on the intrinsic value of personhood. Further, love requires that death not become so commonplace in human thought that the loss of even one is not felt in the deep places of human sensitivity. The dependent relationship of patient upon family and physician is a symbol of every person's dependency upon and responsibility for the other. Thus, love's losses to death are to be taken seriously.

Even so, love also cares enough to "let go" and accept its adjustments to life and living beyond death. Those who have loved someone who desired death instead of prolonged agony know that it can be profoundly selfish to impose the will of the healthy upon the desire of the dying. At times, it is profoundly cruel to keep a patient alive. Love may show its most profound dimension in permitting the beloved to experience the peace that only death can bring. Love, then, requires both resisting and cooperating with death.

One's view of moral responsibility regarding death may also include elective death by "direct and voluntary" means. One may decide to "drink the hemlock" when suffering from disease or illness that is incurable. Choosing to die may require greater moral heroism and a more profound theology of death than succumbing to the coincidental ministrations of medical care after one's own cognitive functions have ceased. Such persons may be seen as acting in the context of Christian freedom and under the burden of personal responsibility for life-and-death decisions. Suicides of this type are hardly to be viewed as sins for which there is no forgiveness. On the contrary, such acts may be based upon the understanding that it is more human and more dignified to die setting the terms with death than passively to await death as if one could neither anticipate nor deal with its coming. Certainly, for the Christian, such an act may signify a commitment to the truth that "whether we live or whether we die, we are the Lord's" (Rom. 14:8). What is of ultimate importance is not the manner of one's death but the responsibility one accepts for dealing with death in the light of the victory of Christ.

Chapter 5

THE BIBLE
AND
BIOTECHNICAL PARENTING

Biomedical parenting involves overcoming childlessness by means of technical intervention. While certain forms of such procedures have been known and practiced for many years, recent breakthroughs in medical science have introduced novel possibilities that bristle with legal and moral issues.

A woman has given birth to a child on behalf of a Kentucky couple. They were childless after many years of marriage. The surrogate, a happily married mother of three, agreed to be impregnated by AI using the contracting husband's sperm. For this service, she was provided a fee roughly equivalent to a salary in the business world for the time she invested. Should such arrangements be morally condemned if not legally forbidden?

Louise Brown was born in 1978—the result of a medical experiment known as *in vitro fertilization.* The mother had blocked Fallopian tubes and thus was unable to conceive. Doctors removed an ovum and fertilized it with her husband's sperm in the laboratory. Then, the fertilized egg was replaced in the mother's womb, where it developed to term. The "lovely Louise" was the result. Are such procedures immoral even though they produced a beautiful child? Thousands of couples have applied for this procedure in America. The first "test-tube" baby has already been born, and six other pregnancies were begun in 1981. Should it be outlawed before it gets out of hand?

An obstetrician sought counsel from a panel composed of psychiatrists, a lawyer, chaplains, an ethicist, physicians, and clergy. The group was composed of equal numbers of men and women. The question: Should the obstetrician use artificial insemination to impregnate a patient? She is in her mid-thirties, single from a second divorce but very much determined to have a baby. After considerable discussion, a show of hands revealed that the panel was equally divided between those who thought he should aid her pregnancy and those who thought it inadvisable.

These cases indicate some of the ways in which people are now able to deal with infertility. Each poses moral questions in different ways. However, the novel factor in each case is that pregnancy is not the consequence of sexual intercourse. Biotechnical means are used to bring about fertilization in each case, and implantation in one. Are such procedures contrary to biblical perspectives on parenting?

If so, they are not directly or obviously opposed by the Bible. Neither are they directly suggested. The world of scientific technology confronts us with problems not dealt with in the biblical story. The means of artificial insemination and in vitro fertilization were not available to our biblical ancestors and thus were not directly addressed. However, there are biblical paradigms and theological perspectives from which principles may be discerned to provide guidance through the maze of arguments pro and con that have been generated.

THE PROBLEM: INFERTILITY

The problem of infertility is as old as recorded history. The Bible records numerous instances of couples who faced the frustration of permanent or chronic sterility. Abraham and Sarah, Jacob and Rachel, Elkanah and Hannah are couples who stood in the long line of frustrated but hopeful couples who have been denied their desire to produce offspring. By definition, infertility is the failure to produce a viable pregnancy within a year of regular sexual intercourse without the use of contraceptives.

The human reproductive system is complex and delicately balanced. Many things can go wrong to interfere with or prevent the central, determining event, the union of male sperm with the female ovum. The Ethics Advisory Board of the Department of Health and Human Services has said that approximately 7 percent of American couples are infertile. Some estimates range as high as 15 percent. This means that 5 million to 10 million people are facing this frustrating barrier to parenthood. The incidence of infertility seems to be increasing. Over the last fifty years the sperm count in American males has dropped over 30 percent—a dramatic decrease by any standard. In 1929, there were 90 million sperm per cubic centimeter; in 1974, this had dropped to 65 million and by 1979 to 60 million. While exact reasons are not known, environmental factors are thought to be a major source of the problem.

A low sperm count does not make one infertile, of course. When the sperm count is unacceptably low, hormone treatments are usually effective. Male infertility may arise from a variety of sources. One is the blockage of conduits through which sperm travel, such as the problem of varicocele, a collection of enlarged veins in the scrotum. Another problem may be a malformed penis that does not deliver the sperm through the tip of the glans and thus hinders the sperm from reaching the cervix. Undescended testicles can also cause sterility unless the problem is discovered and corrected in early adolescence. Some occupations also cause sterility, such as radiation exposure or truck driving that requires long periods of sitting. One man was born without testicles. Only with the injection of testosterone was he able to develop male characteristics or libido. He was made fertile, however, by a surgical procedure that gave him one of his brother's testes.

The success of the surgery made it possible for him to father a child.[1]

Among females, infertility may be traced to a condition called anovulation, in which no egg emerges from the ovary. This may be caused by hypothalamus or failure of the pituitary gland to produce sufficient quantities of hormone to stimulate ovulation. Another hormonal-related problem is that in which the fertilized egg does not receive a hospitable environment in the uterus. The egg dies instead of implanting. For this and other reasons, one scientist has said that probably 25 percent of fertilized ova never implant but are passed through the monthly menses of the woman.[2] Another problem is the absence of or the blockage of the Fallopian tubes. Sometimes scarring from veneral diseases such as gonorrhea blocks the tubes and hinders passage of ova through them. The endometrium, or soft lining of the uterus, may also cause such scarring. For reasons that are as yet unknown this material may move into the abdominal cavity and attach itself to organs such as ovaries, tubes, and bowels. With the monthly cycle, this material expands and crumbles but is not discharged through the vaginal opening. The result is irritation of sensitive tissues, leaving disruptive scars. Other sources of female infertility include fibrous tissues in the uterus and a malformed cervix which cannot resist the weight of a growing fetus. These conditions may be correctable by surgery. A final category relates to cervical function. Normally a mucus is produced by the cervix through which the sperm swim to the awaiting egg. If this mucus is absent or the consistency is too thick, the sperm's passage is blocked. This, too, is treated with hormones.

Infertility created by male and female problems may include timing of intercourse to coincide with ovulation. Sometimes toxins or other antibodies are created by the male or female and kill off the sperm. Stress also seems to be a factor in some types of infertility. Undetermined causes constitute a major category of infertility cases.

The description or analysis of the causes of infertility is one thing. The impact upon a couple is quite another. Being sterile or infertile has a dramatic effect on the self-esteem, self-image, and sexual confidence of the couple. As one person put it, "It is not merely an inconvenience, it is a major life crisis."[3]

Even the "routine" efforts to discover the causes can be a major source of anxiety, pain, and discomfort to the couple. The "problem" may be endometriosis, but it is terribly disturbing to have a doctor announce as he peers through a laparoscope that it is all over your insides. Biopsies of uterine tissue, frequent blood and urine samples, ingestion or injection of hormones requiring repeated office visits and burdensome, if not nearly prohibitive, costs, all become involved in the quest for pregnancy. Years of reading temperature charts and timing sexual intercourse may make the couple forget what spontaneous lovemaking is all about. The hope of corrective surgery may be followed by the despair of more waiting and living through many more menstrual cycles. Even possible corrective treatments are done with the candid admission that science "knows more about how to help couples not have children than how to help them have children."[4]

THE BIOTECHNICAL POSSIBILITIES

Such discouraging news must now be set in the context of new possibilities that are being explored in the laboratories of medical science. Genetic engineering holds out the promise that many, if not most, of the problems associated with infertility can be remedied. As defined by the American Medical Association, the term covers "anything having to do with the manipulation of the gametes or the fetus, for whatever purpose, from conception other than by sexual union, to treatment of disease in utero, to the ultimate manufacture of a human being to exact specifications."[5]

This chapter deals only with interventionist strategies to bypass infertility and enable a couple to become parents. Questions dealing with the manipulation of the genetic material itself will be treated in the following chapter. Already at least eight ways of aiding people to become parents are known. The only nontechnical method is the coital-gestational, which has served to bring the human race to its present genetic state. The others are biotechnical:

Artificial insemination (AI) involves using the husband's (AIH) or a donor's (AID) sperm to impregnate a woman. A physician introduces sperm into the woman's uterus, where, it is hoped, it will fertilize the awaiting ovum. Widely used to improve the quality of thoroughbred livestock, this is now a standard procedure as a way of dealing with male infertility. Probably as many as 150,000 Americans have been conceived by AI. Each year from 5 thousand to 10 thousand pregnancies are begun by AID alone.[6] The sperm may be fresh or supplied from a sperm bank, where semen is frozen and stored.

In vitro fertilization (IVF) involves extracting a ripened ovum from a woman's ovary, fertilizing it in a petri dish in the laboratory, and then returning the embryo to the woman's uterus, where it is hoped the ovum will implant and develop to a normal birth. Already children have been born to couples in Australia, England, and America, and other successful pregnancies have been reported from the General Hospital, Norfolk, Virginia. The process is designed to enable women to bear their own children even though their tubes are blocked. Each child is entirely that of the married couple genetically.

In vitro fertilization has several advantages: (1) It meets the childbearing desire of the woman; (2) the child bears the genetic features of both married partners; (3) there are no risks to a "third party"; and (4) there are no risks of strain between the married partners because of the contribution of another woman who might be perceived as a competitor.

Egg transfer involves transferring an egg from a donor woman to an infertile woman's uterus. The egg then may be fertilized by the recipient's husband.

Artificial embryonation (AE) requires flushing an embryo

from a woman who has been artificially inseminated by a donor's sperm, then implanting the embryo in the womb of the donor's wife. Half the genetic identity of the child will be that of the husband of the couple. The wife contributes the nurturing environment of her womb, though no genetic factors. The Reproduction and Fertility Clinic in Chicago offers this service at a cost between $10,000 and $12,000. It is also planning to offer embryo adoption.

Embryo adoption (EA), or prenatal adoption, involves both donor sperm and donor egg, but they would be transferred to the womb of the recipient and she would bring the fetus to birth.

Ectogenesis is the nurture of a fetus from fertilization to viability in an artificial placenta or glass womb. The human womb is enormously complex and extremely difficult to duplicate in the laboratory. The Italian embryologist Daniele Petrucci claims to have grown an embryo in such a container for 29 days. He destroyed it when it appeared grossly deformed. A repeat experiment resulted in keeping a female embryo alive 59 days. Experiments in America used aborted fetuses—a practice now illegal. Other mammalian fetuses are being used, however, so the technology is still being developed.

Cloning, or nuclear transplant, consists of removing the nucleus of an egg and replacing this with the nucleus of either a donated unfertilized egg or the nucleus of a body cell. The re-nucleated cell is then implanted and brought to term in the womb. The child has only the genetic material of the donor of the nucleus.[7] Since only a male or a female seed is used, this is a process without conception. It is artificial virgin birth—a child with the same DNA as the (one) parent.[8] David Rorvik popularized this term, claiming that a wealthy man had arranged for a woman to bear a clone of himself.[9] The claim sensationalized the subject but was without foundation. There is no evidence that any primate or mammal has been replicated by cloning, though the possibilities are intriguing to many scientists and laypersons. The theoretical know-how is being pursued. The technology is already available.

Monogenesis or parthenogenesis is potentially a still further method. This involves spontaneous embryo development from one gamete or sex cell rather than from the union of two. This occurs in nature chiefly among plants and invertebrate animals. Thirteen species of lizards have only female populations. There are also certain small fish and one type of white turkey that do not use males to produce offspring, which are near duplicates of the mother. Exactly how this happens scientists are not certain. But they do know that the process can also be accomplished artificially, by chemical, electrical, or mechanical stimulation of the egg. It has been done with rabbits, mice, frogs, and birds. Some scientists dismiss as "science fiction" the notion that it might be done among people, while others believe that it certainly will be tried and probably will be successful. Estimates are that it happens naturally among humans about once in every 1.6 million pregnancies.

Surrogate Parenting. The woman who carries the child to term will not necessarily be the mother of the child, of course. She may be a surrogate, bearing the child for another woman or couple who will rear the child as its parents. Alvin Toffler distinguished between "bio-parents," who give birth and genetic endowment to children, and "pro-parents," professional child rearers who tend, love, and nurture the children to adulthood.[10]

The possibilities for biotechnical parenthood in the future are limited only by the imagination. *Cloning* offers the ultimate ego trip—a child made *exactly* in one's image. *Monogenesis* suggests artificial stimulation of the ovum of a single woman who desires children but not sexual relations with a male! The radical feminist or a lesbian couple can engage in the ultimate male-rejection syndrome and still perpetuate "their kind." *Ectogenesis* conjures up visions of embryo factories where babies are grown in glass wombs and are available for purchase at birth by interested persons, whether couples, individuals, or groups. *In vitro fertilization* suggests manipulating genetic material at fertilization so that the genetic characteristics of four or more persons may be passed on to the child.

If these possibilities evoke negative feelings, there are other possibilities that are more positive. *Embryo transplants* offer hope for couples who have chosen to be sterilized for genetic reasons. They may be carriers of recessive genes, such as sickle-cell anemia, Tay-Sachs, hemophilia, or Huntington's chorea, which they do not want to pass on to their offspring. Now they can bring a child to birth that has a better chance for a life without serious handicaps and, at the same time, fulfill their desire for children. *Egg transfer* makes it possible for a woman whose ovaries produce no ova to bear nevertheless a child by her own husband. While the genetic contribution would be from the female donor, the child would be no less that of its mother.

Surrogate parenting offers still other advantages. This novel approach to parenthood involves a woman bearing a child for another woman, one who is presumably infertile. At least three such births have been reported in Kentucky and more are supposedly on the way. In the most famous case to date, a Kentucky couple contracted with an Illinois woman to bear a child for them. The contracting wife could not bear children because of blocked Fallopian tubes. The surrogate, a happily married mother of three, agreed to bear a child for a fee. The woman was artificially impregnated with the contracting husband's sperm. Paternity tests established that it was not the child of her own husband. Even so, it was necessary for the child to be adopted by the contracting couple, since a child belongs to the mother until she signs away her rights under U.S. law.

CONSIDERING THE OBJECTIONS

Such new approaches to human reproduction have raised a number of objections. Some of these are directed at the manner in which sperm is collected (masturbation), at the consequences that will result if such procedures gain widespread acceptance, and at the legal issues involved. A brief account of some of these approaches follows.

Masturbation. All artificial insemination procedures are sometimes condemned because they involve voluntary ejaculation. Masturbation is against natural law and thus constitutes mortal sin, according to traditional Roman Catholic moral theology. Pope Pius XII condemned AI in his 1949 address on medical ethics. For him, AI totally separates procreation from the unitive aspects of sexuality. His real concern, however, seemed to have been with the means by which such sperm are acquired, namely, masturbation.[11]

The biblical basis for this moral notion is the story of Onan in Genesis 38. "Onanism" in older Catholic moral dictionaries is defined as masturbation. Onan was commanded by God to impregnate his dead brother's wife, Tamar, so that his brother would have issue (v. 8). Instead of impregnating her, however, he "spilled his seed on the ground." For his sin, according to the story, God killed him (v. 10).

However, Onan's sin was not masturbation but his refusal to give his deceased brother a child (v. 9). The text is clear on this point. He probably engaged in *coitus interruptus,* but there is no basis in explicit biblical teaching to condemn masturbation. Certainly, whatever moral reservations one may hold regarding masturbation, this text is not a sufficient ground to condemn artificial insemination procedures. The entire point of the Onan-Tamar story was that Tamar *should have been impregnated.*

Logically, those who use this story to condemn procuring semen by voluntary ejaculation would have to advocate the use of adulterous coitus for impregnation. Certainly, the intention to produce a child or to contribute to that end removes such acts from the obsessive-compulsive syndrome of harmful autosexuality. Morally, the act is no different when it is the husband's sperm than intervaginal ejaculation. Bernhard Häring, admitting the uneasiness that traditional moral thought creates, still argues for the rightness of enabling couples to have a child by artificial insemination. As he says,

> We have to see the loftiness of the parental vocation as an essential part of marriage and the immense joy of the husband and wife, who for years have desired children and through this manipulation are now able to receive their own child in an atmosphere of genuine love.[12]

Demystification of Sex. Another objection is that the blending of scientific technique with human sexuality will demystify, deromanticize, and demythologize sexuality. The fear is that sexual functions will become entirely pragmatic. Childbearing will lose its mystique and the artificial placenta will pragmatize the womb. These objectors envision a society in which couples decide on childbearing for economic and social reasons rather than the purely personal calculation of a desire for children. The mystical side will be replaced by the rational. Sexuality will be simply another part of human existence, not a mystery based in awe and wonder.

Toffler saw the emergence of biotechnical reproductive techniques as a result of the flattening of the emotions necessary to accommodate the marketplace.[13] As the family is streamlined to allow maximum freedom for the woman, the mystique of motherhood itself is sacrificed. Jacques Ellul sounds the same note in warning of the desacralizing effect of technique.[14]

The Masters and Johnson studies of human sexual response were opposed for such reasons. As they showed, however, the robe of mystery that surrounds sexuality is frequently no more than a veil of ignorance. Lack of information may contribute to a sense of mystery, but it also creates enormous problems. The widespread incidence of venereal disease, unwanted pregnancies, and sexual frustration among married couples is frequently traceable to the lack of knowledge of sexual function. Ignorance seldom serves human well-being.

Some flattening of emotions is to be expected as science

unravels some of the intricate workings of human reproduction. That unraveling will not be evil but may well contribute to health and realism about our bodies. Too often the church has confused ignorance with morality and superstition with revelation. The loss of such ignorance will be mourned only by incurable romantics, mystics uninterested in sexuality and antitechnologists. But it need not disturb people nourished in the biblical tradition.

We can celebrate sexuality without believing it to be either divine or demonic. Technical intervention can serve to bless us and not curse us by enabling us to better control our procreative powers and facilitate making choices about responsible parenthood.

Contradiction to Permissive Abortion Laws. Some persons point to an irony of the present situation: although there are over a million abortions in America each year, there is a black market in babies. Further, thousands of couples have their names on the waiting lists of adoption agencies. This argument is often pushed to advocate the prohibition of abortions *because* so many couples would like to adopt a baby.

This argument can be answered briefly around several points. First, abortion availability is not the primary reason for lack of adoptive children. There are literally thousands of children available for adoption. The problem is that they are not infants, they are nonwhite, of mixed ancestry, or handicapped. In other words, prospective parents are looking for healthy, white infants to adopt. While that may be understandable, it should be clear that the problem is not the lack of adoptive children.

A second factor in the abortion-adoption ratio is that many women are choosing to keep their babies born outside of marriage. Whereas a decade ago 90 percent of those who gave birth outside of marriage gave the child up for adoption, 90 percent are now choosing to keep the baby. Thus, it is not so much abortion as it is a shifting attitude toward single parenthood that has limited the adoptive infant market.

The most serious objection to this argument, however, lies

in the not-so-subtle suggestion that women should be forced to have babies so others can adopt them. The idea is that compulsory pregnancy is justifiable as a social good. There is considerable moral difference between a woman who voluntarily decides to give her child for adoption and one who is coerced to remain pregnant because someone will adopt the child. The implications of this line of reasoning are frightening. Only a short step remains to the justification of compulsory impregnation *and* pregnancy for the reasons of social demand for adoptive children. The only women victimized by compulsory pregnancy in the Bible were slaves. Their story was not told, however, as to their feeling of depersonalization and lack of respect. They were slaves—without rights or legal recourse. The abolition of slavery was based upon the recognition of its moral bankruptcy. The denial of the right to decide one's own direction in life, including pregnancy and maternity, cannot be tolerated by civilized society. Even through the institution of prohibitive laws, the basic decision of a woman not to be pregnant should not be denied—even for the well-being of others.

Population Control. Groups and individuals concerned about overpopulation often object to biotechnical procedures because they bypass a "natural" check on population growth. Some couch the objection in religious language, claiming that infertility is God's will that the couple not have children. Others are more pragmatic—their concern is simply to limit the birthrate in any way possible. Some use the humanitarian argument. While admitting the dimensions of tragedy and frustration for the couple, these groups in the long run consider population control to be the most humane way of reducing the population growth rate.

The concern for overpopulation is legitimate. Applied to biotechnical procedures, however, the objection is misplaced. Very few couples, relatively speaking, will ever be affected by these procedures. Cost factors, the scarcity of resources, the novelty of such procedures, and a general social and personal reluctance to resort to them, all indicate limited use. Many of the procedures, such as cloning, have not even been successfully used on human subjects. The success rate of in vitro fertilization is extremely low. The number of people added to earth's population through such procedures is not going to account significantly toward overpopulation.

The problem of overpopulation stems from people having too many children, not from the few who desperately want at least one. Population control measures do not need to deny children to anyone. What is needed is that everyone exercise a responsible stewardship of procreative powers.

Commercialization: The Booming Baby Market. Many people see the development of such procedures as an example of the way in which economic forces shape personal choices and the human future. Couples who desire a child are a "ready-made market" for people willing to exploit that desire for commercial gain. People are willing to "buy babies," or "sell babies," or "rent their wombs" for profit. One writer referred to a Reproduction and Fertility Clinic as having "human embryos for sale."[15] Surrogate mothers are referred to as "mercenary."

One unemployed nurse offered to bear a child for a California couple for $10,000. She wanted to get herself and her daughter off of welfare. "My whole point," she said candidly, "is to make some money." When a Michigan couple advertised for a surrogate they had numerous offers. One was from a woman who asked for one year's expenses to medical school. When the offer of money was withdrawn because of the legal opinion that this constituted buying babies, the surrogates also withdrew.[16]

The concern of the courts is based upon the fact that a black market in children has flourished at times. Only recently in Colombia, South America, a multimillion dollar scheme was uncovered which involved selling children. People in Europe were buying children kidnapped or purchased in Colombia, Peru, and Ecuador. Prices ranged from $10,000 to $15,000. The combination of greed, desperation for children, and affluence creates a market the unscrupulous can exploit. The children involved are the helpless victims of uncaring adults who are willing to abduct, abandon, or sell them. One couple recently tried to trade a fourteen-month-old boy for a sports car.[17] Laws to prevent cruelty to children or a traffic in children are necessary.

Courts in Kentucky and Michigan have rendered opinions that surrogate parenting is in fact illegal because of the laws forbidding baby buying. The Michigan court declared that "the right to adopt a child based upon (a) payment . . . is not a fundamental personal right and reasonable regulations controlling adoption proceedings that prohibit the exchange of money (other than charges or fees approved by the court) are not constitutionally infirm." The state's interest, the court said, was to "prevent commercialism from affecting a mother's decision to execute a consent to the adoption of her child." The fear was also expressed that such arrangements threaten the family: "Mercenary considerations used to create a parent-child relationship and its impact upon the family unit strike at the very foundation of human society and are patently and necessarily injurious to the community."[18]

Kentucky's attorney general asked the court to rule the practice illegal under laws forbidding child buying. He pointed out that the woman is not only paid a fee, in addition to medical and travel costs, but must return the fee if she decides to keep the child. Another problematic is the provision under Kentucky law that no consent for adoption may be given before the fifth day after birth. Mrs. Kane had agreed to the adoption even before impregnation.

These opinions will be challenged as to their adequacy or accuracy. Applying laws prohibiting baby buying to surrogate parenting seems a problematic extension of a law based upon a valid concern. Public policy should prohibit couples from selling a child from mercenary motives, whether to aid the remainder of the family to live with greater ease or to get off of welfare. Mrs. Kane was paid a fee, but her motives were hardly mercenary, apparently. Her desire was to let a childless couple know the joy of a child. She enjoyed being pregnant and was healthy and happy.

Furthermore, the child is also the child of the contracting father. He already has certain rights and responsibilities toward the child. Presumably, for instance, should the couple —for whatever reason—refuse to accept the child, the surrogate could sue for child support under existing paternity laws. Contracting for and providing funds to bear one's own child is hardly the same as buying a child. The fees involved are more appropriately described as compensation for an invaluable and risky service rendered. The investment of time, the curtailment of activities, the impact on body and emotions, the threat to the health and life of the woman, the requirements of medical tests (all with added risk), all are recognized as compensatory. The costs themselves are not unlike the expenses involved in other methods of achieving pregnancy. *Adoption* procedures are costly. *Artificial embryonation* costs in excess of $10,000. *In vitro fertilization* is also costly—$3,500 to $4,000 regardless of outcome.

New modes of parenting are bringing new legal problems with which the courts must deal. The old laws on baby buying are the only basis upon which surrogate parenting could be legally tested. It is likely that they will be found inadequate. New legal measures will need to be developed. Mercenary motives and commercial exploitation are a valid concern of law and morality. That problem needs to be rectified in the medical community as well as in the black market, however. Wanting children is neither a crime nor a sin; exploiting prospective parents for greed of gain, even if cleverly disguised as concern for the patient, is an evil to be avoided. In this, as in so many areas of life, "the love of money is the root of all evil" (I Tim. 6:10).

BIBLICAL PERSPECTIVES

Running through religious discussions of biotechnical reproduction are assumptions that need to be examined from a biblical perspective. These permeate the debate on the objections briefly treated above. They are far more complex, however, and thus deserve to be isolated and discussed at greater length. In this area, the issue of the personhood of the conceptus is a primary concern, since germinated cells are being manipulated in several of the procedures. The larger context of the discussion is that of the moral basis for procreation. This will be treated under the subject of a theology of parenting.

Is the Fetus Human?

Objections to biotechnical parenting strategies are most frequently based on concern for the fetus as person. Antiabortion groups have voiced shrill objections to any type of funding for in vitro fertilization clinics, such as that in Norfolk, because of their belief that the conceptus "created" in the petri dish is in fact a person. All fertilized ova that are not implanted they regard as discarded or destroyed persons. This is the genetic definition of personhood which has been discussed in the chapter on abortion.

This notion of personhood has basic flaws and cannot be accepted in the sense of establishing parity or equality of value or rights between the fetus and the woman. Even so, the humanity of the fetus must be taken into account in discussions of biotechnical parenting. This is true because a child is deliberately being brought into being. Not only are there concerns for the health and well-being of the woman, therefore, but also for the fetus.

George Annas argues that the question of in vitro fertilization, for instance, should be answered on the basis of the best interest of the child.[19] His point is that if it can be shown that the risk of deformity is unusually high or if the psychological impact on the child is injurious, then IVF should be discontinued. Morally, children cannot intentionally be brought into the world without due regard being given to their well-being. It is not a matter of only giving a woman a child; it is a matter of concern for the child as well.

This brings the question of the humanhood of the fetus into focus, which might be called anticipatory personhood. The fetus is to be treated with a regard and a concern due a person, because it is being deliberately planned. It is therefore accepted, and anticipated, as a child to be.

Anticipatory personhood should not be confused with actual personhood. The fetus is not a person but should be regarded as such. Those who oppose biotechnical parenting procedures believing that we are in effect creating people in a petri dish make a basic mistake. "What worries me," one doctor said, "is, if I am experimenting, trying embryo transfer, I get to the six- to eight-cell stage and then I deliberately stop that, I'm killing a human life."[20]

Anticipatory personhood is not the same as actual personhood. Those couples who eagerly plan a pregnancy and in hope await the coming of a child into their home and lives will relate to the fetus as a person very early in pregnancy. People eager to be parents will joyfully welcome the news of pregnancy. A new person is on the way! In their talking to the fetus, in their exuberance of this glad news, the child is brought into the circle of the human family. It is *named* a child—called a person—even though it is not yet a person.

Jürgen Moltmann underscores this truth in distinguishing between the *vitality* of the fetus and its *humanity*. The origin of humanness is not so much in biological beginnings as in the atmosphere of acceptance and recognition given by others. He points out that "it belongs to the essence of human life that it is *accepted* and *affirmed, recognized* and *loved.*" The question is one of the value of the fetus to those involved in the family, not one of vital signs. The nurturing, "human" atmosphere of family is essential to the development of the person from the embryo:

> In the moment when the mother, the parents, the family—to name only those most proximately concerned—develop a relationship of acceptance and affirmation for the embryo, the

atmosphere of humanity is established in which this nascent life can become a human life.[21]

One sign of humanness is the ability to include others in that circle of people who are not themselves actual persons. To be human is to treat as persons some who are not persons. Pets are frequently loved so dearly that they are regarded as "one of the family" or as being "just like a person." So the human community extends its boundaries to protect and care for many who are not truly persons. Attributing personhood to them is an important sign of personhood itself.

Rachel Smith, reflecting upon her own pregnancy, recognized that when a child is desired it is not a "thing," nor a mere part of a woman's body. It is another self, a person recognized and given personal standing by a personal self. As she says: "The mother, as the residence for this other being, is filled with a sense of its value, which is apart from her own sense of value. Though intricately bound up with this being, she is distinct from it."[22] Her joy was the celebration of the gift of a child, a person-to-be, whom she could love and embrace as a person.

Attributing personhood to the fetus is a function of the humanity of the parents and others involved who are in fact persons. They know that the beginnings of every individual as person can be traced to that mysterious union of sperm and egg, which begins the process of our development. As persons, we know that our individual life is on a continuum from conception to death and we relish the mystery and power of the beginning as well as the process. Knowing that, we can rejoice in the beginning of new life in the womb.

There are numerous passages in Scripture that convey this sense of anticipatory personhood. They combine several elements: (1) the declaration of God's active involvement in creation, (2) the consciousness of cooperating with God in this creative event, and (3) the celebration of a special moment from God. These are often doxological in nature, joyously declaring what God has done in bringing one into being. Or they may be reflective and devotional, contemplating the purpose of one's being.

Jeremiah is an example of the latter. He declared that God had known him even *before* he had been formed in the womb (Jer. 1:5a). The context of this passage is his account of his calling as a prophet. His credentials for the ministry to the nations (v. 5c) are from God, who has brought him into being for a special purpose. (See also Isa. 49:1–5 for a passage with similar meaning.)

Donald Shoemaker says this passage ascribes personality to all unborn fetuses.[23] This betrays the context and pushes it far beyond its obvious meaning. The passage is highly personal. It is not a rational discourse on how God creates people. Jeremiah declared that God *knew* him, *formed* him, and *consecrated* him. All these support his central claim: God is the reason for his existence and the source of his calling. The claim on the basis of this passage that God causes every pregnancy is no more supportable than claiming that God predestines every person to be a Jeremiah.

Certainly we can affirm God as the source of our being. "In him we live and move and have our being," Luke declared. "We are indeed his offspring" (Acts 17:28). God is the Creator and thus is the power of all that is. The psalmist echoes the same sentiment:

> For thou didst form my inward parts,
>   thou didst knit me together in my mother's womb. . . .
> Thou knowest me right well;
>   my frame was not hidden from thee,
>   when I was being made in secret,
>   intricately wrought in the depths
>   of the earth.
>
>   (Ps. 139:13–16)

The image is that of a person reflecting on the marvels and mysteries involved in the formation process. A parent may ponder the wonders of a child newly born, touching and reflecting upon every tiny limb. The feeling is one of amazement and quiet joy. The religious person will have a sense of awe and gratitude to God for that new life given by God. Parents know that they are not the power of procreation or the source of life. They participate in a power beyond themselves and are part of a process that does not originate with them. Nor do they have absolute control over it. We may be channels of life, cooperators with God in conveying new life, but we are never creators.

Prospective Caring

Thus, any discussion of whether a woman should be impregnated by artificial insemination must include questions as to the well-being of the child. Here the issue must be faced by the medical team as well as by the woman, precisely because biotechnical parenting is a cooperative venture. Certainly the desire to be pregnant is not the same as an absolute right to have a child. Not every person who wants a child is suitable to be a parent. The medical team that is requested to assist the impregnation must consider the environment of nurture and acceptance into which a child will be born. The desire to be impregnated can no more be considered a demand that *must* be met by the physician than a patient's insistence that a leg be amputated without medical indications. Parenting procedures are even more serious morally, precisely because a child will be produced.

The Norfolk clinic, for instance, has been careful to screen applicants so as to select only couples who evidence a stable relationship. The child has a right to be born to parents who are themselves stable and thus will provide a healthy home environment in which the child will be nurtured. This was the consideration that led many on the panel to believe that the obstetrician should not cooperate with the single woman's pregnancy.

Concern for the child-to-be will also weigh the psychological impact of certain procedures upon the child. It can be expected, for instance, that children produced by AID will someday be curious about their donor parent. This is similar to the experience of adopted children who want to know their parents of origin. This does not seem to pose a major problem, however, and thus should not be used to condemn such procedures. It does focus the responsibility for concern at this level and for providing guidance for working through the dilemma when it occurs.

A more important problem is raised by Häring when he deals with the prospect of childbearing by ectogenesis. He considers this a "loveless way" to produce a child and wonders whether such a person would not suffer great damage psychologically in the specific human capacity to reciprocate love.[24] At this point, there is no way to tell, of course. But the question is important. There are profound emotional factors involved in uterine gestation that are important to fetal emotional development. Attempts to "duplicate" the environment of the human placenta will need to incorporate such elements. Until those factors are sufficiently dealt with, ectogenesis will remain morally untenable. The same criterion would apply to the suggestions that human embryos might be nurtured in the uterus of cows so as to relieve women of the maternal burden. Nonhuman environments ought not be used for human subjects. The psychological and emotional development during gestation is important in caring for the humanity of the fetus.

Finally, concern for the child involves scrutiny of the genetic risks involved. Ramsey fears that the risk of genetic deformity from IVF experiments is so great that none should be done. For him, it amounts to experimentation on a human subject without consent. And even if only *one* were severely deformed, the immorality of the experiment would be obvious.[25] He is operating on the assumption of the actual personhood of the fetus, which leads him to such an absolute prohibition.

Certainly genetic risks will be involved. There always are when sperm and egg meet. Already, one surrogate mother has given birth to a handicapped child. The use of donor sperm has also at times resulted in deformed fetuses because of recessive genes. Presumably, however, the statistical incidence of deformity will be no greater through these procedures than through ordinary pregnancy. The insistence on "consent" to be born is absurd. Consent of the fetus is no more required than with any other birth. Children neither will nor request their being brought into existence whether through coital-gestational or through artificially assisted pregnancy.

Where deformities are detected in utero, the persons involved will be confronted with the dilemma of whether or not to terminate the pregnancy. Surrogate contracts in Kentucky require amniocentesis and other tests for genetic abnormality. However, there is no indication of requirement to continue or to terminate the pregnancy should deformity be detected. Presumably, the decision would have to be made on the basis of information available and the word and religious convictions of the parties involved. Should the surrogate and the contracting couple not be able to agree on whether or not to abort, a legal dilemma would be faced. It is not clear whether the contracting couple would still be responsible to adopt or whether the wish of the surrogate has priority. In at least one case, the contracting couple proceeded with the adoption.

Legal entanglements aside, the moral questions at that point involve the same considerations that pertain to the abortion decision. There is no way to say in advance whether the pregnancy should be terminated or not. At that time, the circle of those involved, but most especially the pregnant woman, will face the necessity of decision regarding continued pregnancy.

Due regard for the personhood of the child-to-be will require a concern for optimum genetic health. It would be cruel and unloving to induce pregnancy just for the sake of producing a child. To will a child into being is also to will as nearly as possible to assure the genetic health and well-being of the child. Anything less amounts to abdicating responsibility once the pregnancy has been induced. The willingness to artificially begin a pregnancy should also require the responsibility for assuring optimum health for any child so produced.

Procreation: The Biblical Promise

Discussions of the morality of biotechnical reproduction also involve a theology of procreation. The couple, and more specifically the woman as a moral agent who has both needs and responsibilities regarding childbearing, is here brought into focus. Whether procedures to bypass infertility ought to be used cannot be settled simply by reflecting on the well-being of the intended child. Neither the childless couple nor the physicians who may facilitate pregnancy are setting out simply to create a child. The profound human need to express and extend itself in progeny is the issue at stake. Biblically understood, that need is rooted in creation, the divine promise of procreation and the calling to parenthood.

Creation and Sexuality. The desire for children is rooted in the creation of people as sexual beings. The creation narratives portray man as male and female (Gen. 1:27). The Bible affirms that both sexes bear the image of God and that personhood is inextricably wed to sexuality. The *imago Dei* is not their sexuality, however, for God is nonsexual. People procreate by sexual congress. God creates by the spoken word. The biblical image of personhood can never be separated from sexuality.

Affirming the sexuality of our being does not mean or require that one must be sexually active. A person is male or female and can achieve wholeness and completion of personality whether or not that person is married or sexually experienced. To be sure, the ordinary pattern in Scripture is the active sexual life in marriage. In that bonding of commitment and love, people live in intimate relation to another sexual self. But marriage is not intended for everyone. This is confirmed in the Christian story of the incarnation. Jesus was "truly man" but was apparently celibate. There is no evidence that he was ever married. But that does not diminish his being a sexual person. It does show that personhood is not tied to sexual activity.

Another distinction to keep in mind is the one between the sexual drive and the desire for children. The Bible recognizes the intimate connection between sex and propagation. However, the meaning of sex is not primarily that of procreation. The creation of sexual differentiation and the experience of sexual desire were both recognized as prior to childbearing (Gen. 2:8). Coitus is primarily expressive of love and intimacy, and thus has meaning apart from childbearing.

Those religious traditions that attempt to make sexual interest licit only if it is tied to the desire to bear children distort the biblical perspective. The Bible declares God's blessings upon sexual desire completely apart from the command to procreate (Gen. 2:24–25). Companionship and intimacy are prior to procreation. Only an Augustinian correlation between coitus and a biological transmission of sin can lead to a bias that causes some to seek a moral justification for coitus aside from its pleasure and intimacy.

This tradition also denies the fact that the desire for children will not stimulate sexual interest. The Covenant Code considered coitus basic to marriage (Ex. 21:10). Intercourse was the sign of the marriage bond, sealing the covenant and consummating the vows. Jacob's marriage to Leah and Rachel was signaled by intercourse (Gen. 29:23, 30). Paul's discussion of marriage in I Corinthians 7 argued that intercourse was mutually obligatory between the spouses. Nowhere did he suggest that children were a necessary part of marriage or a moral justification for intercourse.

Sexuality and Procreation. The person is not simply a "free spirit"[26] but is a psychosomatic whole. Mind, body, and spirit are integrally related. The procreative urge is not simply "what one wants" or "desires," as if these were purely rational or emotional ideas. It is rooted in biology—in the evolutionary heritage we have as creatures of earth. Sexual inter-

course is not just the attraction between the sexes. It is also
the primeval urge to procreate. Sexual intercourse is both
pleasurable and procreative. As procreative, every particular
act of coitus does not need to intend pregnancy as part of the
stewardship of procreative powers. Certainly, after the desire for children has been fulfilled, that capacity might be
permanently removed by sterilization. But that does not
alter the fact that sexual intercourse is procreative. Coitus is
both the symbol and the primary means of pregnancy and
procreation. This biological component cannot be removed
from definitions of personhood without doing serious damage to the biblical notion of person as a psychosomatic whole.

This rootage of procreation in biology has important meanings for women considering surrogate parenting. Women are
not simply machines able to develop products without serious attachment to the product itself. A bonding relationship
is established during pregnancy which is both biological and
psychological. The woman's chemistry alters, there is the
interrelationship of two unique systems—the greater dependency of the fetus is met by the maternal need-dependency
of the woman. This is the meaning of symbiosis (*sym*—"with"
or "together"; *bios*—"body")—bodies living together for mu-
tual advantage.

Any woman who gives up a child (as for adoption) is literally giving away a portion of herself. The child is the extension of the self—the embodiment of one's extended self. At
least one possible meaning of the biblical notion of *henosis,*
or "one flesh," is that it refers to the offspring of the sexual
union (Gen. 2:24; Eph. 5:31). From the two—the man and
woman—comes the one, the child who is both them and not
them. They are intricately bound up with the being of the
child and yet are distinct from the child.[27]

The trauma of separation from the body in birth is in part
a biological response to loss of bodily ties. As new or altered
chemistry begins, the perspective and outlook of both
mother and child are affected. Where the child remains with
the mother, the adjustment is facilitated by the social and

personal interchanges possible between the two. Where it is disrupted by the removal of the child, the trauma may be more severe.

Early in her surrogate contract, Elizabeth Kane felt she could give up her child without seeing or holding it. The contract specified that she would do neither. The child was to be delivered directly to the waiting arms of the contracting woman. At birth, however, the need for seeing and touching was too great to resist. With permission, Mrs. Kane did both. Not surprisingly, another surrogate has changed her mind and decided not to give up her child to the contracting couple.[28] That any number of surrogates would have a change of mind and heart is entirely predictable. Women are not unfeeling machines. What began with the objective resolve of a clinical or even commercial contract moves perceptibly and inevitably to a question in which the whole person is involved. One does not part with a child as if one were writing a check.

This also points to the dynamics behind the shift among women pregnant outside of marriage. Nine out of ten of those who bring their pregnancy to term are now keeping their child. The personal relationship of mother to child can be accommodated in response to powerful social ostracism, but given a more favorable social climate, women will predictably opt to retain the child.

This also has relevance for the abortion debate. Those concerned that every woman confronting a problem pregnancy or an unwanted pregnancy will choose to abort have not taken this important bonding into account. Very strong reasons of social circumstance, personal well-being, or threat to health are usually necessary for the pregnant woman to set aside her maternal experience. Nature has a strong impulse toward preserving itself and perpetuating its kind through pregnancy and childbirth. Not only the anticipated joys of having children but powerful biological impulses are at work in women who are willing to literally risk their lives to bear children. Unless and until that genetic detail is removed from personhood itself, the perpetuation of the human species through coital-gestational birth will be assured. Terminating pregnancy—for whatever reason—denies a factor basic to our humanhood. This is why abortion is never an easy matter for the woman, confronting her with her own humanness and its linkage to others in an unavoidable way. The decision to be pregnant or not to be pregnant is profoundly human and religious. One is confronted with the Creator and with human relationships to his work. This does not settle the moral question of abortion, of course. But it does point to the gravity of the choice.

Spiritualizing the Procreative Need. Recognizing the psychosomatic nature of personhood also means that the temptation to spiritualize the problem of infertility should be resisted. Richard McCormick opposes IVF, for instance, saying that such procedures subtly redefine love "in a way that deflates the sexual and bodily and its pertinence to human love."[29] The comfort-counsel he offers those frustrated by infertility is to recognize the New Testament stress on relationships of commitment which are more important than biological needs. He notes that Jesus defined family membership in terms of moral values and spiritual perceptions rather than biological ties (Matt. 12:46–50; Mark 3:35). He cites John the Baptist's statement to the effect that "the children of Abraham" are people of faith characterized by repentance. God, John said, could create children from stones if natural origins were all that were important (Matt. 3:9; Luke 3:8).

McCormick correctly notes that the nature of faith in the Bible transcends all biological definitions. The apostle Paul defined our ties to Abraham in terms of faith, not biological ancestry (Gal. 3:7). Adoption was another favorite metaphor of Paul by which he related God's action in creating a family or community of faith (Gal. 4:5; Eph. 1:4-5).

The truth of these passages is basic to a Christian understanding. However, they offer neither guidance nor comfort to the couple who desperately want a child. Such desires cannot and must not be treated as if they are solely emotional dilemmas that can be satisfied by greater spiritual depth. For most people, prayer is not a satisfactory substitute for progeny.

Far from such texts being used as arguments against IVF, they may well support an even broader range of biotechnical procedures. The imagery of adoption is vital to surrogate parenting, prenatal adoption, and embryo transfer. In each case, the child involved must be accepted by a parent who has no biological or genetic ties to the child. If acceptance of parenting responsibilities and the ties of parent to child were premised primarily on genetic ties, such procedures should never be used. At that point, considerations pertaining to the well-being of the child would be operative. If that child could not be loved and fully and unreservedly accepted as truly a part of the family unit, it would be immoral to bring that child into being. However, the human experience shows that children can be accepted fully and devotedly when adopted by a couple who chooses them in love. This is the human paradigm of God's acceptance of us who are adopted into the household of faith.

The Promise of Offspring. A further biblical theme important to biotechnical parenting is God's promise of procreative power to his creatures. Here a distinction is necessary between the promise of procreation and a command to procreate. Genesis 1:28 has God saying: "Be fruitful and multiply . . ." This is often interpreted as a commandment indicating they *must* have children. The context of the story indicates, however, that this is more accurately interpreted as *promise.* You *may* have children. Certainly, God did not set forth a universal requirement. Jeremiah chose not to have children. Jesus and Paul chose singleness and celibacy. If procreation were God's *command,* they were disobedient. The truth is that they were acting in the freedom of permission granted by God pertaining to offspring. Those religious interpretations which have regarded this as a *command* have contributed to overpopulation and human misery. This was not the purpose of God.

The Bible regards children as a divine blessing. The pleasure and companionship of intercourse may also produce the added joy of a child. This is not only the pleasure of a new person who enters relationship with mother and father. It is also the joy of participating in the power of ongoing life. Sometimes this was thought of as the person living on through the life of their descendants. This probably accounts for some of the extraordinary ages accorded some of the Old Testament figures. A great man's age was calculated as the sum of the ages of his direct descendants.

An even more profound cause of that joy, however, was the recognition that the couple is cooperating with God in bringing new persons into being. This awareness is symbolically portrayed in the renaming of the woman. She is no longer to be thought of as "woman," the she-man. Rather, she becomes Eve, the living one, the mother of all (Gen. 3:20). Creation has become procreation. God's work in fashioning his creatures is seen also as empowering those creatures with the ability to perpetuate their own kind (Gen. 1:12, 22, 28). All living things become co-creators with God. That biblical declaration adds depth, beauty, and profundity to the role of childbearing. Thus, while there is no *requirement* that every person be a parent, humanity is permitted to cooperate with God in perpetuating the human species.

The promise of God has the dual dimension of cooperation with God and continuity through offspring. These are dramatically embodied in the story of Abraham and Sarah. Through their own experience of delayed fertility, they learned their radical dependence upon God for the power of procreation. Only God is the giver and power of life. They were not the authors of such power but desired to share in its wonder. Abraham seemed to have expressed primarily the desire for an heir. He wanted a son to continue his work. The son would bear the covenant promise to future generations. Sarah desired to bear the fruit of her own body. She is a paradigm of every woman who desires motherhood. A woman's biology both is and is not her destiny. Not every woman wants or should have children. For those who want a child of their own, however, nothing is more important. Destiny and personhood are related to biological function.

The Bible and Infertility

Infertility is both a personal frustration and a theological problem, therefore. At the personal level, the woman is unable to act out her sense of calling to motherhood. This creates a crisis in personal well-being for the couple, but especially for the woman. The unfruitful wife in the Old Testament was "the embodiment of need and misery and abandonment," says Karl Barth.[30] Hippocrates observed that "many and various are the ills of barren women." The deep longing for children can lead to various psychosomatic complaints. A person's entire life can become consumed by the quest for a child. One's salvation in God cannot be complete as long as mind and body are so burdened.

Objecting to a "managed pregnancy" (IVF) as immoral because it is not therapeutic seems to miss this point entirely.[31] A child is not just another gift or a medical corrective to a physical limitation. A child is a unique gift, comparable to no prosthesis whatever. A child is the gift of person and an extension of the sexual self. For those who desire parenthood, nothing is more "therapeutic" than having a child. The desire can become an obsession affecting every facet of one's life. This is truly a state of unhealth. The well-being of the whole person is at stake.

The distress of Hannah (I Sam. 1:5–18) is a sign of the agony of every wife who desires motherhood. She felt social ostracism (vs. 5–6) and a despair that led to tears and loss of appetite (vs. 7, 10). She petitioned God in fervent and persistent prayer to remove her barrenness. That prayer was granted "in due time" when she "conceived and bore a son" (v. 20). Even the name of the child was testimony to her feeling that he was a special gift from God (v. 20).

Exactly why Hannah was unable to conceive we can only speculate. Some women have thought themselves infertile and proceeded to adopt a child only then to become pregnant. Perhaps a similar change in body chemistry or psychological outlook took place with Hannah. But she regarded it as little short of miraculous. Her relief from barrenness was a bondage broken—a sign of the salvation of the Lord (2:1). This is why the knowledge of becoming or being pregnant is an occasion of pure joy for those committed to motherhood. Linda Lynch (not her real name) shrieked for joy when doctors at the Norfolk clinic told her she was pregnant.[32] Her joy was not unlike that of Sarah (Gen. 21:6) or Hannah (I Sam. 2:1). These women, separated by generations and centuries, were united in their sense of being that was so closely tied to their drive for motherhood. They shared the same joy of the Lord when that need was granted.

The child induced by biotechnical means is, then, no more depersonalized than were Isaac or Samuel. Each child was a gift of the Lord—truly miracle births.

This story also portrays *infertility as a theological issue.* The intention of God in creation and redemption is frustrated. His intention is that people be able to experience the powers of procreation and engage in the procreation of life. This is both the special gift and the promise of the Creator. However, a malfunction in the bodily processes prevents the fulfillment of that promise of God—that hope of the couple.

Promise and Paradigm. Having a child was of enormous importance in the Old Testament. The patriarchs thus went to considerable lengths to overcome infertility. The experience of Abraham and Sarah (Gen. 16:1–5) is a biblical paradigm of surrogate parenting. They had heard the promise of God that they would have a son, but Sarah was apparently infertile. When she was seventy-five, and convinced she would never become pregnant, she took Hagar, her maid, and presented her to Abraham, that he might have a child. The text indicates Sarah's feeling that "I shall obtain children by her" (16:2). Sarah declared that the surrogate's child would in fact be hers!

A similar story is that of Jacob and Rachel. Though Jacob

had children by Leah, Rachel was apparently barren. Thus, she presented her maid Bilhah to her husband as a way of giving him children (Gen. 30:3). With both Sarah and Rachel, bearing a child was an important factor in their marriage and in their sense of personal fulfillment.

Another provision that underscored the importance of childbearing was the levirate law. Deuteronomy 25:5–10 required that, should a married man die before he had children, a surviving brother should impregnate the widow. This would be the child of the deceased. The story of Onan and Tamar in Genesis 38 is based on this law. Onan's refusal to impregnate Tamar was regarded as the sin for which God slew him (Gen. 38:10). The story served as a powerful enforcement to Hebrew men to carry out the responsibilities of the levirate law.

Undoubtedly the Hebrews were also concerned to keep their women from marrying outside their group. It was extended to the "next of kin" (Ruth 4:8) when there was no surviving brother, as in the story of Ruth and Boaz (v. 10). Here the concern was not only children but property and inheritance.

Such biblical paradigms certainly do not establish the moral acceptability of biotechnical reproductive procedures. They do indicate how important childbearing was to the biblical family, however. So strong was this desire that creative options were employed to bypass the frustration of sterility. On this basis the principle can be established that infertility as such was not regarded as the will of God which must be passively accepted. If handmaids were an acceptable means of realizing God's promise, it seems reasonable to believe that the Hebrews would certainly have been willing to use the far more humane means of artificial intervention.

Infertility and Divine Providence. Some have argued that the will of God is found precisely in the biological blockage. Some notions of divine providence link "nature's way" with God's action. Thus, if the woman is infertile, God wills that she not have children. Any action to overcome her infertility would therefore violate the will of God.

However, the providence of God can in no way be inferred from just anything that takes place in nature. We can no more conclude that God makes some women infertile than that he directly causes people to be born blind (John 9:1–5). The mistakes of nature contradict the will and intention of God. To be sure, there are Old Testament passages that indicate the belief that God caused barrenness (Gen. 20:18; I Sam. 1:5). The assumption was that sin was related to infertility. This compounded the grief of those women who could neither account for any sin nor receive the evidence of forgiveness. In cases such as those of Sarah and Hannah, the curse seemed arbitrary, if not capricious.

They had no medical explanation for infertility. Rather than search for "causes" in scarred tissue, hormonal imbalances, blocked Fallopian tubes, or malfunctioning ovaries, they explained infertility as the action of God. This theology held that both good and evil proceeded from the first and only cause of everything (Isa. 45:7).

Contemporary Christians have a twofold advantage over their biblical ancestors. First, we have the advantage of medical science that gives explanations of bodily functions. We are not condemned to seeking supernatural explanations for whatever happens in nature. Secondly, the revelation of God in Christ clarifies once and for all the nature of God as one who is love (I John 4:7). As loving Father, "God works for good in everything with those who love him" (Rom. 8:28).

Science and the Stewardship of Parenting

This establishes an important biblical principle for dealing with the moral acceptability of biotechnical reproductive procedures. God *works with* people to accomplish his will and bring about his intention for their lives. This is the biblical perspective which gives religious support for medical science and its efforts to enhance longevity, stronger bodies and minds, and the control of disease.

Scientific knowledge or technical expertise facilitates work in cooperation with God, using the resources that God has provided in nature for the well-being of the human community and the natural environment. Technology and science should not be viewed as enemies of God and humanity but as facilitators of faithful stewardship. Spiritual interests and moral purposes basic to the biblical view may be served by science. What is needed is a venture in partnership rather than a conflict over territory between science and religion.

There is no biblical support for the notion that whatever is "natural" is "godly" and whatever is "artificial" is "ungodly." The biblical view is rather that anything may be used for evil purposes or for good. God is the source of all wisdom, including that which makes it possible to enhance human well-being and serve human need. People are those unique creatures who are able to contrive techniques and construct technologies to bring about better health and stronger bodies.

People are not creators. They work with the "givens" of God's creation. Ramsey seems to miss this point when he decries in vitro fertilization as "a manufacture by biological technology."[33] Those physicians who manipulate sperm and egg to produce a pregnancy do not in fact "manufacture" anything. The power of impregnation does not belong to physicians—they are engaged in a cooperative venture with God. They wed technical skills to nature's processes, placing the biological materials in a favorable environment where sperm, egg, and uterus can begin and continue the work they are designed to do.

Joseph Fletcher overstates the case when he says that "the more rationally contrived and deliberate anything is, the more human it is."[34] For him, "it is precisely artificiality which is man's hallmark."[35] On this basis, he can approve of biotechnical procedures without reservation:

Laboratory reproduction is radically human compared to conception by heterosexual intercourse. It is willed, chosen, purposed and controlled, and surely these are among the traits that distinguish *Homo sapiens* from others in the animal genus, from the primates down. Coital reproduction is, therefore, less human than laboratory reproduction.[36]

The truth to which he is pointing is that it is a uniquely human ability to use artificial means to assert dominion over the harmful effects of nature. However, he fails to acknowledge two important facts. First, biotechnical parenting is not entirely artificial or nonnatural. All the material used is entirely natural, as is the gestation process. Even an artificial placenta would have to imitate the natural processes of a female uterus to a minute detail. Thus, at most, the procedures under discussion are a manipulation of natural materials by human intervention.

The second omission in Fletcher's optimism is the recognition that rationality and deliberation can also be used in inhumane ways. Uniquely human powers may be used to destroy uniquely human values.[37]

This is the concern that prompts Ramsey to condemn such procedures entirely. While he could approve corrective surgery for the "clinical defect" causing infertility, he says that procedures like IVF are morally unacceptable.[38] Enabling a woman to have a child of her own is a praiseworthy therapeutic objective, he says. However, the spheres of marital lovemaking and procreation are not to be separated. Using means other than coital-gestational involves interchanging human procreation with manufacture. He fears that science is trying to move life's beginnings from sperm to term entirely into the laboratory. The end result will be that society totally separates procreation from coitus. He sees Huxley's Hatcheries in the not-too-distant future.

If Fletcher is too quick to approve, Ramsey is too quick to condemn. Disapproving of artificial means just because they are artificial places a cloud of moral doubt around any medical procedure. All of medicine is interference with natural forces. However, it is not antinatural or nonnatural, since many of the substances used mimic those found in nature.

The "pill," for instance, is a chemical contraceptive utilizing sex hormones to stimulate or create a false pregnancy, thus suspending ovulation.

Human medicine bridges the world of the natural and the artificial. Physicians use technical means to correct bodily malfunctions. Many natural processes are inimical to human well-being. Infant mortality, pernicious anemia, and hemophilia are all "natural." The religious community is unanimous in saying that medicine should cure these if possible, however, for they contradict the intention of God that people should be healthy. Infertility is also natural. It is also inimical to human well-being and thus contrary to God's intention.

Thus it cannot be wrong in principle to use technical means to bypass a biological or physiological barrier to parenthood. Enabling people to become biological parents is one way that nature is modified and, at the same time, fulfilled. By modifying the "natural" function of a woman's body, the natural longings for childbirth may be realized and nature's way of perpetuating the human race can be facilitated. As long as it is natural to have and want children, it cannot be unnatural or unacceptably artificial to facilitate the process by medical science.

CONCLUSION

At this level, biotechnical parenting has a symbolic value that brings together several biblical principles. First, it points to the goodness and rightness of sexual intercourse on its own. Coitus is not primarily for procreation but for the expression of intimate love in the context of marital commitments. Secondly, the love of the couple may be served by their deliberate choice to become parents. Choice, not chance, governs this pregnancy. The child is assured of caring love from the very first. God's intention for every child is thus symbolized. Finally, parenthood is related to calling, not to accident or mere biological capacity. Emotional and

spiritual commitments to the tasks of parenthood are far
more important than the relatively simple process of giving
birth. Those who confront the frustration of childlessness,
who weigh the commitments that may and will be required
and are willing to invest time, energy, devotion, and considerable financial outlay to become a parent, symbolize the
consideration and commitments that are integral to the biblical sense of calling. These are parents by design, intention,
and purpose. They will recognize their child as the extraordinary gift it truly is. They will not resent the pregnancy as an
untimely accident or reject the child as an unwelcome in-
truder. Every child should be as fortunate. To such commitments every parent is called.

Chapter **6**

GENETICS, THE BIBLE, AND THE HUMAN FUTURE

Humanity is confronted with a genetic crisis. For all the hopes generated by the beneficial discoveries of medical science, it often appears that as many problems have been created as have been solved. Lurking behind the scenes of the grand victories and public disclosures of new discoveries there is a specter few people dare observe and many refuse to confront. The problem is that of the genetic future of humankind. The basic building blocks of our bodies and brains seem to be in jeopardy.

The Elephant Man is a story of human tragedy that dramatically portrays the issue. In both the stage and the movie version, the story of John Merrick has been told with insight and sensitivity. Merrick suffered from neurofibromatosis (Von Recklinghausen's disease) which afflicted him with huge scales and lumps that developed from the bony tissue of his body. A mystery to his physicians, he was a curiosity to the public, who subjected him to ridicule and frequently treated him as a circus freak.

This is one of the most common inherited neurologic disorders. Approximately 100,000 people in the United States have the disease, which affects all areas of the nervous system and skin. Benign tumors appear on the brain, spinal cord, and skin. Vision and hearing are affected. Merrick's disease symbolizes the plight of millions of people around the world. Genetic illness is an enigma to scientists and a source of pain and limitation for those so afflicted. Such stories of anguish are far too common.

A couple in their late twenties have just experienced a miscarriage. The fetus was deformed, with multiple anomalies. This was to be their second child. The first, a little girl now five years of age, is hospitalized, a victim of severe mental retardation. The couple are at a loss to understand the deformities in their children. The wife is determined not to be pregnant again unless she undergoes amniocentesis and has the option of abortion.

The birth of a little boy to a couple brought joy and excitement. But every time he is touched he screams with pain and his skin blisters and breaks. He has a rare skin disease —dystrophic epidermolysis bullosa. It strikes about one child in 50,000. There is no cure.[1]

A British couple plan to have their three children sterilized. The mother, thirty-three, has Huntington's chorea, a chronic disorder of the nervous system that causes progressive muscular and mental deterioration over a period of ten to twenty years and ends in gruesome death. She had watched her father suffer and die from the disease and knows that her children have a 50-50 chance of contracting it. In order to stop the vicious cycle of passing the disease to future generations, they have decided to end their family line.[2]

The Genetic Burden

These stories illustrate dramatically a further dimension of concern in the realm of genetic engineering. The previous chapter explored the possibilities of enabling infertile couples to *have* children. An even more complex question pertains to the genetic endowment of people. While science has made great strides in medical advances, diseases and handicaps that are inherited remain a source of frustration largely beyond the control of current medical practice. The extent of the problem can be briefly summarized.

Birth Defects

Birth defects loom as one of the most serious problems. Every thirty seconds a deformed child is born. The National Foundation for the March of Dimes says that 7 percent of all babies born in the United States have genetic defects detectable at birth or within the first year of life. These range from harelip to anencephaly. Twenty percent of these 250,000 babies have defects that are caused solely by genetic factors. Sixty percent represent a combination of genetic and environmental factors and the remaining 20 percent are solely environmental. Some of these severely limit the person's mobility or ability to find fulfillment or effectively to serve society. Others doom the individual to an early death or a lifetime of illness. Some are so severe that lifetime hospitalization is required.

Some genetic defects are not obvious. They may be chemical imbalances or nervous disorders that cause severe problems months or even years after birth. Tay-Sachs appears within the first year and typically causes death by the age of three. Huntington's chorea, or chronic brain syndrome, causes death from neurological breakdown, but its onset is delayed until adulthood.

Over one million persons are hospitalized annually as a result of birth defects, while fifteen million cope daily with the effect of such defects on their lives. Medical science now knows of over three thousand human diseases that are genetically determined. This does not include those traceable to environmental factors such as the drug thalidomide. The statistics are alarming: 1 percent of all babies born have an abnormal chromosome; 25 percent of all conceptions are lost through spontaneous abortion, usually because of genetic abnormalities in the conceptus; one of every five sperm or eggs produces a mutation; every pregnancy carries a 3 to 6 percent risk of involving a major birth defect. Excluding accident or injury, 40 percent of the deaths of children in hospitals are traceable to diseases that are genetic in nature.[3]

Genes and Illness

Increasingly, genetic factors are being linked to illness. In some cases, the linkage is established, as with Huntington's chorea. More often, suspicions have been raised but not proven. Cancer remains a mysterious disease in many ways partially because of its complex varieties and partially because its causes have eluded investigators. Genetic factors are invariably suspected, however. It is known, for instance, that Philadelphia chromosome is linked to chronic leukemia. This is believed to be an acquired chromosomal abnormality, however, rather than one that is inherited. Renal carcinoma, a type of kidney cancer, seems to be an inherited genetic abnormality, on the other hand. One family had ten members affected over three generations. Chromosomal studies revealed that three who had a particular abnormal exchange carried an 87 percent chance of developing renal carcinoma by the age of fifty-nine. This is alarmingly high when compared to its general incidence in the population of 1 in 1,000.[4]

A California geneticist claims that he has isolated the gene in humans that could be a cause of mental depression, chronic alcoholism, and even multiple sclerosis. Dr. David Comings, of the City of Hope Medical Center, found that a particular gene was twice as prevalent in people who died of suicide and alcoholism as in the brains of people who died of stroke, heart disease, cancer, or accident. He designated the gene Pc. 1 Duarte. It was found in men and women, blacks and whites. It is a mutant gene different from any others found in the brain.[5]

A relationship between genes and environmental factors in causing disease is also recognized. A woman with type A blood taking oral contraceptives is five times more susceptible to blood clots than women with other blood types. Higher levels of the digestive enzyme pepsinogen 1 in the blood makes one five times as likely as others to develop peptic ulcers. On the Island of Sardinia, a link between hemolytic anemia, the fava bean, and a deficiency of the enzyme G-6-PD was discovered. This explained why some Sardinians were unaffected by the bean, while others suffered lethargy or death from contact with or eating the fava.[6] In such cases the genetic factor is exposed by the environmental. Disease results only when the two are brought together.

Genes may also produce *resistance* to certain diseases. High levels of H D L (high-density lipoproteins) reduce the risk of heart disease. Ironically, sickle-cell anemia produces resistance to malaria.

Longevity itself may be tied to genetic factors. Many scientists believe the body cells contain a type of biological clock or genetic timepiece that is related to life expectancy. When the "clock" runs down, the person dies. Researchers are attempting to discover the secrets of this clock so it can be reset or slowed down. That, theoretically at least, would be a breakthrough enabling people to live beyond what is now normally possible.

Behavioral characteristics are also traceable to genetic factors. Clear and provocative evidence now exists that criminal behavior may be related to the makeup of the autonomic nervous system. A study of twins and adopted children, conducted at the University of Southern California and New York University, indicates that children whose fathers were criminals were more than twice as likely to become criminals themselves even though they had no contact with their natural parents. The study involved 1,145 males in Denmark who were adopted between 1924 and 1947. Doctors theorize that the makeup of the nervous system may account for callousness, lack of remorse, inability to learn from experience or punishment, failure to anticipate consequences of certain acts, and seeming inability to "feel." Definite differences were detected in the measurement of certain areas, such as skin conductive tests, pulse rates, chemical levels in the blood, and brain-wave patterns. The tests suggest that the nervous system is different, if not deficient, in those with criminal behavior.[7]

Such studies go beyond the theory that relates an extra Y chromosome (XYY) to a tendency toward violent behavior. Here the search is for significant neurological or metabolic abnormalities. Some of these might be caused by environmental factors such as injuries, but others may be traceable to genetic makeup. That bodily chemistry affects behavior is rather widely known. Personality differences may be traceable to glandular organization and regulation. Underactive thyroids cause lethargy; overactivity causes one to be excitable and high strung. Overactive pituitary glands can produce nymphomania.

In sum, our genes carry not only physical but behavioral characteristics. They shape every part of the person's physiological and psychological makeup. This is underscored by the development of mind-altering drugs, especially the hallucinogens which simulate psychotic states of mind. Such possibilities make more plausible the theory that mental illness itself may result from inborn errors of metabolism. Psychiatry increasingly relies upon chemistry for the treatment of mental illness.

Deterioration of the Gene Pool

Of major concern to a number of geneticists is the deterioration of the gene pool. That is, genetic weaknesses are being spread to ever-increasing numbers of the population. Some estimate that the number of children born with genetic deficiencies will double in the next five to ten generations. The incidence of Down's syndrome among boys increases nearly 10 percent from generation to generation. The number of girls affected is much smaller, but the rate of increase is about the same.

Those with observable or obvious problems are only the tip of the iceberg. Many others carry recessive disorders. Each person carries a "genetic load" of five to ten defective genes. David Lygre estimates there are at least a hundred people who are carriers of a disorder for each one who is affected.[8] The trend for the future is that both the numbers of people afflicted and their proportion to the overall population will increase. Genetic pollution is a time bomb, slowly ticking away.

George Kieffer argues that gene pollution is a public health hazard.[9] Certainly genetic illness is debilitating and communicable. Like an epidemic, it is spreading harm throughout the populace through the introduction and multiplication of bad genes.

Calculating the Costs

The burden created by genetic problems both for individuals and society is enormous. The toll in human life and potential is practically immeasurable, for it goes beyond economic calculation. Nor can it be limited to those directly affected, for the problem is shared by family, friends, and society. The misery, frustration, and pain are intangible but nonetheless important factors in the burden borne by the afflicted.

Other costs involve the vast outlay of public and private funds to care for those with genetic handicaps. The most seriously afflicted require hospitalization and total care from birth to death. Presently, at least one fourth of all hospital and institutional beds are occupied by persons who suffer from genetic illness or malfunction.[10] The United States spends $1.7 billion annually to care for those institutionalized from Down's syndrome. Annual treatment for a person with Tay-Sachs is about $25,000; and hemophilia about $15,000. Kidney dialysis, provided by the U.S. Government, now costs nearly $2 billion per year, far in excess of predictions when the program was begun.

Such costs will increase in the future. One factor will simply be the inflation of medical costs. The other will be the expected increase in the number of persons requiring care. As techniques to manage genetic errors become more sophisticated, more people will be kept alive and more carriers will produce more people with gene-related disorders.

Koop describes one child born with multiple anomalies, the primary problem being that of ectopia cordis, the heart outside the chest. Fifteen different procedures over a period of 1,117 days were required to reposition the heart and allow for adequate function of the lungs. After this lengthy hospitalization, the child was cared for in the home, where he continued on a respirator. No financial statement was made, but one can surmise that the total costs were staggering.[11]

RESPONDING TO THE PROBLEM

The picture that emerges is one in which literally millions of individuals are suffering from genetic illnesses or handicaps and the human race itself is in a state of genetic decline. The prospects for the future are rather grim. Even if the percentage of genetically handicapped people remains constant in relation to the population as a whole, the numbers of carriers of such diseases are bound to increase. To this point, according to the Hardy-Weinberg theory, once a mutant gene enters the population, it remains at an equilibrium. Thus, the percentage of people afflicted remains the same even though the number of people afflicted greatly increases because of population growth.

However, with better medical care at the euphenic level, carriers will live longer and thus produce other carriers. The equilibrium has been possible thus far in part because of natural selection. Infants with phenylketonuria (PKU) will lead relatively normal lives with a carefully controlled diet. The gene they carry, however, will show up in their children. Hemophilia, also controlled at present, shows up in the male children of those women who are carriers. Genetecist Arno Motulsky has calculated that the frequency of this disease will increase from one in 14,000 to one in 7,000 in less than a hundred years.[12]

A second factor working against the equilibrium is that of mutation caused by environmental factors. New genetic defects are being created constantly. Lederberg has estimated that 80 percent of our mutation rate comes from environmental factors for which people are responsible.

Even the thought of accepting an equilibrium as an acceptable rate of genetic handicaps seems to reflect a moral cynicism. Neither science nor religion can live comfortably as long as vast numbers of people are so afflicted. The vastness of the problem, the intensity of personal anguish, and the extensive costs—both in loss of creative human contribution and in terms of economic resources—to society are problems that cry out for relief. The plain truth is that there can be no possibility of an actual reduction in the number of those affected by genetic disease without some type of medical intervention.

Strategies of Response

There are three type of strategies for dealing with genetic defects. *Euphenics,* which deals with biological improvement after birth, involves optimizing the health and functions of people by modifying or controlling the effects of harmful genetic endowments. This is basic medical treatment. Insulin aids diabetics to live relatively normal lives. A regulated diet prevents serious mental retardation from PKU. Blood transfusions *in utero* save Rh babies. Such treatments are therapeutic aids for individuals afflicted by a mistake of nature. Certainly research and new developments are welcomed and encouraged on the basis of our concern for human health and well-being.

However, such treatments do nothing to prevent genetic ailments. Nor do they offset the negative effect of passing on such genetic details to future generations. By giving extended life and added strength to such persons, future people will be similarly afflicted. The gene pool will carry a greater burden. The morality of intervening at the treatment level poses moral issues in terms of its impact on future generations.

Eugenics, the science of improving the qualities of the

human race, is the second type of strategy to reduce the incidence of genetic defects and improve the human gene pool. This proposes to deal with the problem by careful mate selection and responsible birth control. Presently, of course, these efforts must rely on the education of the public and the general awareness of couples regarding their genetic responsibility. Over two hundred genetic counseling centers are available in the United States to provide guidance.

Couples faced with the knowledge that their children are likely to have genetic defects have several alternative courses of action. One is to *proceed with childbearing.* According to a doctor at Massachusetts General Hospital, about one out of six couples who are told of the risk go ahead with the pregnancy; another New England study reported that two out of six couples were undeterred by the bad news.[13] The will to propagate one's own is so strong that no risk seems too great to bear. According to one genetic counselor, "Couples . . . knowing that they have one chance in four of having a seriously defective child, and that two out of four of their children are likely to be carriers, still frequently take a chance that things will turn out all right."[14] Sometimes a pregnancy is begun with a commitment to undergo tests of the fetus *in utero* to determine possible defects. This is especially true if there is a good chance of having a normal child.

Presently there are no laws in the United States that would require high risk couples to give up sexual reproduction. The presumption is that couples are free to reproduce regardless of their genetic traits. Some physicians cooperate to keep such knowledge a secret from a person the patient is about to marry. Joseph Fletcher cites the instance of a South Dakota family that spread a genetic disease by keeping it a "family secret." The problem was an incurable dominant gene defect causing ataxia, or spinocerebellar degeneration, a progressive loss of speech and muscular control. Its onset comes in the late twenties (thus after marriage and children are born) and takes fifteen to twenty years to run its course before death. The National Institutes of Health had also kept a lid of silence on the case until 1970 when one family's physician requested that the facts be made known.[15]

Another alternative is to *choose contraception or sterilization.* Here the choice is to voluntarily forgo pregnancy and childbearing. Some of the people in the South Dakota case had been sterilized. For Ramsey, this is the method of choice in an ethics of genetic duty. Arguing that couples have no absolute or unqualified right to have children, those who know they have inheritable genetic difficulties should "undergo voluntary sterilization, use three contraceptives at once or not get married."[16] He cites such cases as Huntington's chorea, diabetes, cystic fibrosis, achondroplasia, some forms of muscular dystrophy, PKU, and Tay-Sachs (amaurotic idiocy). For him, a couple's insistence on their right to have children under such circumstances is to betray selfishness and narrowness of vision. Such egocentrism thinks only of immediate desires and does not calculate the well-being of the child or that of future generations.

According to the Agency for International Development, about 65 million couples worldwide have chosen sterilization, which is now the foremost means of birth control. This includes those who want to control fertility as well as those concerned about genetic difficulties.[17]

Eugenic considerations pose the question of personal freedom over against the common well-being; or the right of people to make their own choice regarding procreation over against the right of society to protect itself against the enormous "costs" of supporting the genetically handicapped. Some support the concept of compulsory sterilization for genetic reasons. In Denmark, for instance, marriage licenses are denied to those who carry genetic defects until at least one of the partners has been sterilized. Many states have laws that permit compulsory sterilization of "incompetent" people. Over a period of fifty years, thousands were sterilized in Virginia under a state law that permits such action on a patient "afflicted with any hereditary form of mental illness or retardation," and the procedure is judged "in the best interest of such patients and society." The law had been upheld by the U.S. Supreme Court in 1927. "It is better for all the world if instead of waiting to execute degenerate offspring for crime, or to let them starve for their imbecility," said Justice Oliver Wendell Holmes, "society can prevent those who are manifestly unfit from continuing their kind." The majority opinion continued by referring to the test case before it, that "three generations of idiots are enough."[18]

While such laws remain on the books in many states, they are rarely invoked or applied. The Supreme Court declared one state's law unconstitutional under the Ninth and Fourteenth Amendments in 1942, thus making all such laws constitutionally suspect if not legally infirm.

The problem with compulsory sterilization laws is that they have led to serious abuses of personal freedoms. Premature judgments about a lack of mental competency have resulted in sterilizing people who later showed normal levels of intelligence. Some states have used such laws as birth control measures among blacks and welfare recipients. In North and South Carolina welfare recipients (primarily black) faced sterilization as the price for having their babies delivered.[19] The specter of the genocidal uses of sterilization by the Third Reich is a reminder of the severe abuses to which such practices can be associated. Such injustices are often used to argue the "wedge theory" that any compulsory sterilization is therefore unacceptable.

The problem remains, however, in that narrow corridor of human experience where those who are severely retarded are also permitted to procreate. Unable to make decisions that are "free and informed" regarding their procreative process, ought such persons to be free to marry and have children of their own? The "option" of contraception or sterilization is not even a viable alternative for such people, since such choices require reflective intelligence and deliberate planning. They are the victims of instinctive drives that perpetuate human misery.

A third alternative proposed for couples with genetic defects is that of *artificial insemination by donor.* The late geneticist Herman J. Muller advocated "genetic progress" by encouraging couples to choose to have children of genetically superior people. Recognizing the widespread practice of using AID to overcome infertility, Muller argued that the primary concern should be with the eugenic potentialities of such donor sperm. Sperm and ova banks could be established from which couples could choose in those cases where either partner carries or has a strong chance of carrying some grave genetic defect or where the couple wants to have a child of outstanding ability or vigor. Such banks would not use donor material for at least twenty years in order to note the achievements and quality of offspring of the donor. Such germinal choice, or eutelegenesis, he felt was "the most practical, effective and satisfying means of genetic therapy."[20]

To his credit, Muller attempted to avoid all overtones of racial or class prejudice. He advocated that such programs would be purely at the prerogative of the couple, that careful records be maintained, and that couples have the best professional care available in the fields of psychology, medicine, and genetics. His optimism regarding human nature led him to believe that "this golden chance" would be grasped by couples who "are idealistic enough to *prefer* to give their child as favourable a genetic prospect as can be obtained for it."[21]

Several problems have been raised by critics of this proposal. One is the problem of "the selfish gene"—people want to perpetuate their own genetic material. The "enlightened altruism" Muller counted upon runs counter to the instinctual procreative urges. It is not likely that enough people would ever choose such an option to significantly affect the genetic future of humanity. A second problem is that one would suppose that couples who had the foresight, altruism, intelligence, and vision that would be required to make such a selfless decision would be the very type of persons Muller had in mind to improve the human race. These would, by his own criteria, be the very couples who should reproduce! The final problem is that there is no evidence to support the notion that outstanding people tend to have equally outstanding children. The genetic burden carried by every person means that a handicapped child may be born to any family. Chance combinations produce both unexpected and, at times, highly undesirable results. The problem is illustrated in the now-famous story of the suggestion by the beautiful dancer, Isadora Duncan, that she have a child by George Bernard Shaw. "Just think," she purportedly mused, "a child with my body and your mind." Shaw declined, however, observing wryly, "But suppose it had my body and your mind!"

The problem of the genetic deterioration of the human species therefore remains. Whatever solution is found must be able to deal with: (1) the predisposition of people to want to perpetuate their own self; (2) the insistence on freedom of choice—the individual prerogative above social or political control; and (3) the problem of randomness or chance in genetic combinations that result in illness or handicap. This is why the question in genetic engineering constantly returns to the problem of being able to manipulate the genes themselves. The problem is one that includes both achieving a change in *mores* or religious and personal outlooks that would encourage or accept new means of germinal choice, and the development of the techniques or means themselves.

The Genetic Prospect

Genetics is the third type of strategy for dealing with the crisis of germinal inheritance. This attempts to alter the genes themselves both to prevent birth defects and perhaps to alter the genetic endowments of humanity itself.

For millions of years, natural processes have controlled changes in nature and all living species. Creation is not static but is a continuing and complicated process. The process of each kind producing its own kind (Gen. 1:24) or the emergence of new forms of life may involve a single event or require countless steps over hundreds of centuries. The cockroach appears to have remained the same for a quarter billion years. The prokaryotes, organisms that have no nuclei, have been around for 3.4 billion years. However, for every species that now exists, five hundred have disappeared. Others have undergone tremendous changes, as in the case of the elephant.

A new era has dawned, however. Science now is on the verge of being able to direct changes and thus to a degree control the processes of nature. With the discovery of DNA, we seem to be entering an era of participatory evolution.[22] In people, evolution has not only become conscious of itself. Nature may now be altered by planned design and the creative interventions of this noblest creature in creation. Knowledge of the processes of nature and of the working details of the transference of life now gives people the power to manipulate those processes.

Major breakthroughs in genetic knowledge have taken place in recent years. Mendel first suggested the notion of "units of heredity" in 1866. Less than a century passed before these units were being studied and manipulated. Watson and Crick in 1953 determined the structures of the DNA molecule which consists of two long strands of molecules twisted around each other. DNA is the chemical record of hereditary information. Interlocking strands of DNA constitute genes which are the basic building blocks of an individual's mental, physical, and moral traits. Genes in turn are distributed along the length of the chromosome, 23 pairs of which are found in each of the trillions of cells in the human body. The particular arrangement of these chemicals determines both the species of the organism (whether fish, fowl, or human) and particular features, including intelligence, color of eyes and hair, body form, and sex (male or female).

The combination of chromosomes from the mother and father determines the characteristics of their offspring. The child bears almost equal contributions from each parent. Genetic defects are caused when even one of the thousands of genes is misplaced, abnormally arranged, or damaged. Sickle-cell anemia, for instance, results from a single amino acid variation. The enormous complexity and the billions of combinations or variations possible in such genetic linkages help us to understand why the system frequently results in unfortunate defects in our children.

Nature's processes are characterized by changes and mutations, of course. Some of these are positive and result in stronger bodies and even higher or more sophisticated forms of life. We are all mutants, as Ramsey reminds us.[23] However, many of these changes persist because of medical intervention. They are thus passed on from generation to generation. Each successive generation of people can only be sustained or kept alive by medical intervention, however.

Awareness of the injuries caused by deleterious genes makes intervention desirable. Knowledge of the process of inheritance makes intervention possible. Recent breakthroughs in genetic studies seems to herald the day of being able to manipulate our inheritance factors. The increasing sophistication of computer technology extends the ability to manage the programming details. The precision of microsurgical techniques brings the day of gene surgery, gene deletion, gene insertion, and gene copying ever nearer. The hope that genetic handicaps can be eliminated by genetic intervention does not seem to be an impossible dream.

Studies in recombinant DNA, for instance, have already made certain types of genetic engineering a reality. By splicing genetic material from one organism to that of another a new organism altogether is created. Desirable characteristics from one organism can be transferred to another. Such genes are now creating *insulin* for the treatment of human diabetes; *somatostatin,* a rare brain hormone useful in treating diabetes, gastric bleeding, and other hormone disorders; and *interferon,* which some regard as a breakthrough in treating cancer.

Gene-splicing techniques have already been used in the treatment of hereditary disease among people. Two women, afflicted with a disease in which their bone marrow produced blood cells with abnormal hemoglobin, had normal cells produced in bacteria by recombinant DNA techniques injected into their bone tissue.[24] The procedure, carried out by an American scientist, was highly controversial, since it did not have prior approval for application to people.[25] Even so, it heralds a new era in the treatment of hereditary disease.

The principle involved in artifically producing genetic changes has therefore been proven. All that remains is the technical information to manipulate the tremendously complicated details in the human genetic structure. That is no small step but one that seems certain to be achieved. As Fletcher says, "For the first time in the evolution of life, a living creature [man] has both the understanding and the ability to design itself and its future."[26]

THE BIBLE AND THE GENETIC CRISIS

But ought such intervention to be done? Granted that the plight of those afflicted cries out for artificial relief, the very prospects of altering the genetic features of the human race conjures up images of a "grave new world."[27] The stakes are high, for the future of humankind is involved. As Moltmann observed, "Our knowledge of the stars is a matter of indifference to the stars themselves, but our knowledge of man is not without consequences for the very being of man."[28]

Two currents in history are creating a crisis for humanity. The first is being produced by genetic deterioration, the second by advancing technology. Both are having and will have dramatic effects upon humanity. As Ramsey says, "The crisis of our present-day civilization is genetic at least in part, and one that goes to the very *humanum* of man."[29]

Precisely how humanity is being affected and what responses are appropriate are areas in which there is considerable disagreement. Differences in opinion are not in terms of whether one group is concerned about people and/or the picture of humanity. Both opponents and proponents of genetic engineering seem committed to protect human well-being. Their differences lie in respective answers to various questions. These include: (1) the nature of human person-hood—is it a finished product to be preserved or in the process of development and thus still to be achieved; (2) the relationship of God's providential sovereignty to the natural process, including the evolutionary development of people; (3) the respective spheres of action that are appropriate to people and those reserved only to God; and (4) the question of human stewardship of the process of nature. These are obviously interrelated. The two most critical factors in the debate are the assessment of the threat posed to humanity and the theological perspectives as to divine providence and human stewardship regarding the future of humanity.

Opposition to Genetic Control

Those who object to scientific intervention into biology reflect a fear of the consequences they foresee or they believe that such endeavors are sinful efforts to "play God" and thus should be forbidden. Several of these focus on the impact of technology on the future of humankind.

C. S. Lewis, for instance, opposes genetic intervention as *a threat to humanity itself.*[30] He sees more to be feared from genetics, pharmacology, and experimental embryology than from the abuse of political power or the threat of nuclear destruction! The point of his concern is positive genetics—the alteration of genetic detail to such an extent that humankind will disappear. John Batt sounds a similar alarm in saying that the object of genetics is really man farming. "They don't want to waste their time modifying the behavior of people created by a pair of potentially inferior human beings," he says. "They plan to make their own people. And they are serious!"[31] For them, human nature *as it is* is not to be altered. The human being is not an appropriate subject for such alteration by design. As Lewis puts it, we should not "do to minerals and vegetables what modern science threatens to do to man himself."[32]

A related concern is that scientific knowledge *concentrates power in the hands of a few.* "Technology is power and power is never neutral," as Moltmann observes.[33] For those alarmed about genetic engineering, the future portends an era in which a few will dominate the many. This may be by political power concentrated in the hands of the genetically elite or by mass-producing people who are genetically programmed to be content with their predetermined place in society. The future most to be feared is that Orwellian world of cyborgs and chimeras designed to do their job and no more. This is a world of human predeterminism. The loss of freedom is the loss of humanity: "They are not men at all: they are artifacts. Man's final conquest has proved to be the abolition of man."[34] This is not to be rationalized in the name of man's dominion over nature. As Lewis argues, "What we call man's power over nature turns out to be a power exercised by some men over other men with nature as its instrument."[35]

Further objections are based on the fear that *harmful pathogens may be created* artificially for which there is no immunity or cure. Widespread death and illness could result from recombinant DNA experiments. The potential hazard of such technology is multiplied by the mixture of motives born of desperation or design on the part of the misguided or "mad" scientist.[36] The parallel is to be found in the realm of nuclear physics. Unlocking the secret of the atom has resulted in the possibility of nuclear annihilation. A similar result may happen from DNA experiments. The power to reshape the basic codes of nature is plainly dangerous to the human race.

Those who believe that God's providential work is tied to the processes of nature argue that genetic experiments are *an intrusion into the sphere of God's activity.* People are "playing God" by seeking to overturn what God has done or to create people artificially. This argument is encountered in any experimental work that may even lead to tampering with the genetic codes, as in opposition to biotechnical parenting procedures. As one scientist put it: "There is an old German expression that, roughly translated, means 'One shouldn't poke one's nose in God's affairs.' Let's hope we are not doing that."[37] Thus, genetic engineering is not only hazardous, it is impious—a lack of faith in God. "To tamper with the genes seems to me to 'outrun' God into the unknown future and to exercise an 'elective' discrmimination mere men do not possess," argues Henry Stobb.[38]

Forbidden Knowledge?

This line of reasoning is often extended to include the concept of *forbidden knowledge*. That is, there are some secrets of nature that are reserved by God. People are forbidden to know these things. To do so by research or design is to willfully defy the declared will of God. There are some things that "we cannot morally get to know," Ramsey argues.[39]

This he applies both to knowledge gained by experiments that may result in damage to the person and to research into nature's secrets.[40] From this perspective, the ethical question is whether scientists are morally prohibited from unlocking the secrets and thus altering the domain of nature at the level of a person's genetic endowments. This would be for science a moral equivalent of the legal prohibition against "breaking and entering."[41]

The biblical story to which this appeals is that of the "forbidden fruit" in Genesis 2 and 3. God commanded the man, saying: "You may freely eat of every tree of the garden; but of the tree of the knowledge of good and evil you shall not eat, for in the day that you eat of it you shall die" (Gen. 2:16–17).

Human curiosity and will to power, combined with the subtlety of the tempter's suggestion, caused the couple to transgress the Creator's command. In classical theology, this is known as the Fall, or the first sin of the human race. By that act, evil entered the natural world, and every person is born a sinner. Following Augustine, this tradition posits a primeval "garden" of perfection in which there was no evil. Rational and conscious control of everything from sexual powers to the world of nature was available to the man and woman. Adam and Eve were immortal, they did not age, they had complete control over bodily passions and had infallible moral insight. All these blessings are now lost to people because of the Fall.[42]

That there is evil and sin in the world few people doubt. And few would disagree with saying that there are some ways of getting knowledge that are immoral. The Nazis learned how long people could survive in frigid waters by throwing Jews into icy seas. The immorality, however, was in the way in which they went about gathering the information rather than in the knowledge itself.

Basing an absolute moral prohibition on certain types of knowledge upon the Genesis story is extremely problematic, however. The argument against scientific or technical knowing is more Promethean than biblical. Prometheus was the tragic Greek Titan who stole fire from heaven and gave it to mankind. In his vengeful wrath, Zeus chained Prometheus to a mountain, where an eagle tore out his liver by day, only to have it grow back at night. Zeus was jealous of his divine prerogative and thus tortured Prometheus for intruding upon his territory.

The real issue lies in ignorance, not in knowing. Knowledge is power, to be sure, and can be used for good or ill, to bless or injure, to heal or hurt. But ignorance has no redeeming power or social value. Its most benign face is in that innocence which cannot and does not know. That is found in the subhuman created order that does not have the capacity for discerning the difference between what helps and what hurts or how to use even dangerous knowledge to aid others.

This seems to be suggested in the biblical story of the forbidden fruit. God commanded that Adam and Eve not eat of the tree of the knowledge of good and evil (Gen. 3:3–6). Being tempted to be "like God, knowing good and evil," however, was an attraction that could not be resisted. That knowledge was both a gift or creation of God and an area of life for which humanity is held responsible. The tree of knowledge was created by God and set in the midst of the garden (Gen. 2:9). Forbidden, it was nonetheless "good" because it was created by God. In possessing such knowledge, the man-creature may appropriately be said to bear the image of God. This is godlike knowledge.

The movement of the story is from the "innocence" of ignorance to the awareness of guilt. That knowledge was not technical but moral or spiritual. Humanity was a creature that was aware or knowing in a way distinct from all the other creatures of earth. The story has both progressive steps in the emergence or "creation" of humankind and is a composite of the features that characterize this complex creature. Beginning with the declaration of God's intention to create human beings "in our image" in Gen. 1:26 the story unfolds the various facets of that image in succeeding stages. This creature begins in being fashioned from the same dust as all other creatures. *H'adama* is formed from *h'adam* (Gen. 2:7), as are all the other creatures. The final triumph of this emerging, developing pair, however, is focused in their experience of moral awareness. Their uniqueness is discovered even in disobedience. The disobedience of animals is amoral but that of humans has moral dimensions. They may know the difference in obedience and disobedience and ascribe moral meaning to that knowing.

The emergence of the person, therefore, is signaled in the story of disobedience. Prior to that stage, they are, like all other animals, "innocent"—and ignorant—even of their innocence, much less of their guilt. The dawn of humanity within history happens with the emergence of intelligence and conscience—of rational being that is also morally responsible. This creature is one who makes choices based upon rational and moral considerations.

"Knowing" is awareness. Having knowledge of good and evil is being aware of the moral dimensions of human experience. It is the experience of conscience and of moral meaning. The biblical story of the Fall is a movement from pre-moral consciousness to a new level of intelligence that includes the ability to raise questions about ethical issues. In that sense, it is a fall upward. What is "lost" is the state of innocence and ignorance. Few people would will a return to that "prior" existence. That is to betray a desire to have no moral awareness—no conscience. It is to will away the bicameral mind and to return to the intellectual level of "Lucy," our 3-million-year-old ancestor.[43] Her brain was too small to be that of a human being, but she walked upright and thus had begun the evolutionary journey from innocent ignorance to knowledge of guilt.

Sin and dignity are thus related in the human experience. Where there is no sin, there are no human beings. The dawn of sin awareness is the emergence of *Homo sapiens imago Dei*. Prior to the knowledge of sin and guilt there were no people. Thus to will away our awareness of guilt is to will away our personhood.

The Sin of Ignorance

Sin is involved in the suffering that continues because no one has the knowledge to prevent it. Every untimely and unnecessary death is a sign of the sin of ignorance in the human race. Countless numbers of people died of smallpox before a vaccine was discovered. Some people resisted Jenner's vaccination against smallpox in the late eighteenth century arguing that "if God wants us to have smallpox we shouldn't complain." Had those scientist-researchers drawn back from their investigations because of some moral fear of "forbidden knowledge," people would still be scarred and dying from smallpox. The fault would lie in ignorance—the failure to discover and investigate till cures are found. What science presently does not know may well be the curse—not what it does know. Having opened the world to the atom and unleashed its power, science needs now to increase its knowledge until it can *control* that ominous power. The biblical promise is that of dominion which requires not only knowing *that* but knowing *how* and thus governing processes so as to assure that they are used to benefit, not destroy the human race and/or the world of nature.

One way to understand the presence of disease in nature is to consider it a challenge from God. God's "command" is that people pursue knowledge until ignorance no longer reigns, subjecting people to the futility of unnecessary suffering. Paul seems to suggest that much of the pain and distress of the creation is traced to the ignorance and negligence, i.e., the refusal to know, of people who have not found cures which are "there" to be discovered. He declares that the groanings of the present world are awaiting the revealing of the sons of God (Rom. 8:22–23). Creation will not suffer as extensively when people accept the burden, challenge, and responsibility of knowing. Such knowledge is an extension of human personality into the realm of technique. People are tool makers and designers precisely because they image the powers of God. Technical knowledge is a basic ingredient in being human and indispensable to the tasks and goals of human stewardship.

The Moral Dilemma

Knowing how genetic endowments affect human well-being and being able to calculate the consequences of allowing such problems to multiply make the moral dilemma unavoidable. Concern for the individuals so afflicted and for those persons yet unborn and unconceived who will be handicapped, and a desire to see stronger, not weaker, persons in the future, seem to mandate a response that is itself ethical, namely, to do all we can to ameliorate those problems. The geneticist Theodosius Dobzhansky posed the issue pointedly. "If," he said, "we enable the weak and the deformed to live and to propagate their kind, we face the prospect of genetic twilight; but if we let them die and suffer when we can save or help them, we face the certainty of a moral twilight."[44] His point is that good morals require that we do all we can to help people afflicted with genetic problems. But good morals also require that we care for and protect the gene pool. The awareness that we jeopardize the health and well-being of future generations is a moral dilemma that cannot be ignored. As custodians of the powers of the present generation, we are also responsible for the legacy bequeathed to future generations. It is morally irresponsible to condemn people of the future to a "genetic twilight," the era of such radical and extensive infirmities that the human species is threatened with extermination.

Human Nature and Genetics

Genetics focuses the nature of man as a creature who is retrospective and prospective. People are able to reflect upon their past knowing something of the history and process that God has used to bring them to the present. They are able also to anticipate the future. Both from the biblical revelation and from extrapolations from their awareness of history past and present, they can project the future. Their knowledge of evolution informs them of how God has fashioned the world through millennia of historical epochs. This awareness of the past also says something of the future toward which the world is moving. The future is always an extension of the present and the advent of something new. People can anticipate a great deal and predict a great deal even with considerable accuracy. But they cannot know precisely what the future will bring. We can only know "in part," or partially. The more distant that future is, the less we can predict the specifics. Thus, we can predict that spring follows winter but we do not know the precise date of the last freeze or the first day of 100° temperature. Regarding the population explosion, we can know that, given *present rates of growth,* there will be 12 billion people on the face of the earth by the year 2020. What we cannot know for certain is what may happen meanwhile—widespread famine, nuclear holocaust, or lethal environmental pathogens that may kill millions of people. Or people may awaken to the disaster that such demographic projections portend and take action to avert such catastrophe by instituting population control measures.

The latter possibility focuses the uniqueness of personhood in the biblical perspective. This would be man made "in the image of God," deciding to take action based upon the future *he is able to anticipate.* Of all the creatures of earth, only people can make decisions to avert a future catastrophe or develop a more comfortable, livable future. This requires a combination of intellectual and moral capacities. Reflection and anticipation should result in action that is moral. Knowing the difference between good and evil (Gen. 3:5), people can choose the good and avert the evil.

However, this is not *guaranteed* in the sense of an assured future no matter what we do. God does not determine the outcome by overruling every contrary or sinful act of humanity. People must work with God, not against him, if the future is to be a blessing and not a curse. Thus, Jacques Ellul, in spite of his pessimistic appraisal of human nature, concludes his grand study of technology and its evils by declaring that God's future will be "an extraordinary synthesis of man's work adopted by God and the work of the Spirit brought to perfection."[45]

This is a vital perspective for decisions regarding genetic engineering. The genetic catastrophe lurking in the future of the human race is a challenge for us to *act upon the basis of what it means to be human in order to avert the catastrophe of becoming what humankind was not intended to be.* Only in this way can humankind respond *as person* to the knowledge given to human beings at this juncture in history.

BIBLICAL ESCHATOLOGY AND GENETIC APOCALYPSE

Paul Ramsey rightly sees the relationship between the genetic apocalypse envisioned by scientists and a Christian view of the world. He cites geneticist Herman J. Muller's vivid portrayal of the genetic cul-de-sac into which the human race is heading. Within a few million years, says

Muller, "the then existing germ cells of what were once human beings would be a lot of hopeless, utterly diverse genetic monstrosities." But long before that, the job of ministering to infirmities would come to consume all the energy that society could muster, leaving no surplus for general or high cultural purposes.[46]

He warns that people would have "to live carefully, to spare and prop up their own feebleness to soothe their inner disharmonies and, in general, to doctor themselves as effectively as possible." The time he envisions is one in which everyone is an invalid. Should they have to live under primitive conditions, they would be unable to survive. Only a complex hospital system in that civilization could assure continuity to the human species. The process of genetic deterioration would have reduced them to creatures unlike us, their forebears: "Their only connection with mankind would then be the historical one that we ourselves had after all been their ancestors and spouses, and the fact that their once-human material was still used for the purpose of converting it, artificially, into some semblance of man." The time is foreseeable when "even the most sophisticated techniques available could no longer suffice to save men from their biological corruptions."[47]

The genetic future of humanity is an issue in which biblical theology and science plainly overlap in their interests. Ramsey dramatically and insightfully recognized the points of correspondence between the apocalyptic fears of geneticists and Christian eschatological expectations. He rightly saw that the issue at stake is the manner in which one consciously perceives and intends the world and its future.[48] While he acknowledges the apocalyptic portions of Scripture, he drew back from developing the theme. Instead, he turned the question to a problem of an "ethic of means." The principles he uses to deal with genetics are: (1) that procreation should not be separated from coitus; and (2) that treatment for genetic ills should only be therapeutic for the individual patient.[49] He thus concludes that scientists ought not to intervene genetically. To do so would "only mean the abolition of man's embodied personhood."[50]

The main problem with Ramsey's discussion is precisely that he does not deal with biblical eschatology. He imposes a theological perspective based upon creation. His assumption is that *man as he is* has been made that way by God and we have been told not to tamper with his creation.

The Bible and the New Humanity

Humanity is not a finished product in the biblical perspective. True man is always an eschatological concept. We are not what we once were and are not now what we shall become. On this both science and the biblical revelation concur. Our past is a long and arduous history that moved from simplicity to complexity. But the present is only a moment in time, a new step on a venture of growth and development. We know as little of what we shall become as we do of what we have been. The future holds mysteries yet to be unraveled and vistas of discovery of the personal self for which we have only glimpses of insight. The apostle Paul, speaking of what is yet to be revealed, declared that "now we see in a mirror dimly" (I Cor. 13:12). Moffatt paraphrases this as "the baffling reflections in a mirror."

This is often interpreted as a reference to the limited understanding that people have of God. However, mirrors are for viewing reflections of the self. Paul is speaking of the imperfection of knowledge that belongs to humanity. But he is anticipating the day when self-knowledge will be complete: "Now I know in part; then I shall understand fully, even as I have been fully understood" (I Cor. 13:12). Human life has a *telos,* an ending or a goal toward which it is moving. That goal is wholeness, maturity, or perfection in the sense of completeness. This promise-command is also found in Jesus' statement "You, therefore, must be perfect, as your heavenly Father is perfect" (Matt. 5:48). The term rendered "perfect" is *teleios,* meaning complete or mature.

This movement or process toward the future for humanity

is captured in the biblical notion of Second Adam and Second Advent. Both serve to underscore the eschatological dimensions of being human and, at the same time, provide images by which we are to think of what it means to be human. The "second Adam" of which Paul speaks in Romans 5 is Christ, who is true man. Christian anthropology is Christology at its core. Christ is the norm by which what it means to be human is to be measured. This is why all definitions of what it means to be human can never end with Adam and the Genesis account of the sin of mankind. Genesis is important ultimately only in the light of Christ. We understood human fallenness and imperfection or incompleteness precisely because of our knowledge of Christ. "Man's essential and original nature is to be found, therefore, not in Adam but in Christ," says Barth. "In Adam we can only find it prefigured. Adam can therefore be interpreted only in the light of Christ and not the other way around."[51]

Christ defines what it means to be a person made in the image of God. Still he defies every effort at explanation or description. The mystery of Christ's being is a sign of the transcendence that belongs to every person. The person is always more than the sum of his parts empirically described or scientifically analyzed. This defies explanation, but it can be experienced and it must be respected. In this resides the moral value of personhood.

This means several things for a Christian understanding of personhood. First, it undermines all efforts to provide a fixed or static definition of humanness. Certainly those which focus almost exclusively upon biological functions are inadequate. Neither a particular genotype nor phenotype can suffice as the norm for Christian anthropology. Nor can conceptions like "image of God," or "life," or "breath" drawn from the creation narratives fully suffice, important as they are.

Personhood as we know it is impartial and incomplete—it has a telos that is not yet fully comprehended or experienced. Thus, any working definition of the human must avoid the error of using a static model which is drawn from the past.

The future is just as, if not more, important to our understanding. We are not yet what we are to become. Any lesser
definition condemns mankind to a state of arrested growth.
In short, we will never become what we are intended to be.
As Gustafson says, "Finding what is the human is an ongoing
process of discovery."[52]

Thus, it is false to claim that we have a norm or model for
human personhood that should be preserved against genetic
experimentation. Both individually and collectively, human
beings are changing and developing. There is a process and
a providence at work that is moving toward a future that will
be as radically different from the present as the present is
from the past.

This makes Ramsey's charge that genetic tailoring would
be a "violation of man" terribly problematic. His model for
the human being is drawn from the past (or some imaginative prototype from the present). He has no eschatology in
which the very being of persons participates. His talk of the
future seems little more than apocalyptic rhetoric or a liter-
ary device employed for dramatic effect. This ends by absolu-
tizing a particular portrait or model of the human. This
model is then used as an unchanging, static image which is
not subject to modification at any point. Such a static view of
human nature does not correspond to the biblical portrait of
the person "on the way" to the ultimate realization of God's
will for human life. In short, Ramsey has no eschatology of
personhood.

Second, the Second Adam provides a proleptic experience
and knowledge of what it means to be human. Christ was not
so unlike us that we can never be like him. He is the prefi-
gurement of what humanity is and will be. As John put it
strongly: "We are God's children now; it does not yet appear
what we shall be, but we know that . . . we shall be like him,
for we shall see him as he is" (I John 3:2). What we are and
shall become is always to be measured against the revelation
of God in Christ. Our experience of Christ is a sign of what
is yet to come. "The fact of the new humanity, established in

and by the second Adam," says Paul Lehmann, "means that all behavior is a fragmentary foretaste of the fulfillment which is already on the way."[53]

A third meaning is that the Christian orientation is toward the future, not the past. Both John and Paul are dealing with the future of humankind. Our past is important only in the light of the future toward which we are moving. As Lehmann says, "The Christian lives neither by his 'academic' past nor by his 'Christian' past, but by the future, of which his present is an exhilarating foretaste."[54] The past is not to be discovered in order to be preserved. It is to be understood in order better to relate to our future. This is always the basic thrust of the biblical message. It is a movement from Eden to the Heavenly City, from the Old Jerusalem to the New Jerusalem. This is the story of God's action in history. He moves from creation to redemption, from old creation to new creation, from old humanity to new humanity.

This eschatological perspective is important to the Christian understanding of salvation. While it is correct to speak of salvation as a present experience, it is not true to speak of it as fully completed. Rather, it is a process that has a beginning, a continuity, and an anticipated consummation. As E.M.B. Greene points out, Paul envisioned salvation in three tenses: as a past experience, as an ongoing process, and as a future hope.[55] In this insightful interpretation, he draws not only upon the tense involved in the Pauline texts, but upon the future expectations which the apostle includes in the drama of redemption. The salvation of God awaits the redemption of our bodies, prefigured in the resurrection of Christ (I Cor. 15:2–23). The promise of God is that we shall have a new body, beyond our ability to describe but one of God's own choosing (v. 38). It will be imperishable (v. 42), a spiritual body (v. 44), not made from dust (v. 47) but made in "the image of the man of heaven" (v. 49). Paul admits he is speaking of a mystery beyond his ability fully to grasp or express (v. 51) but affirms that this dimension is an indispensable and integral part of the Christian understanding of humanity and the future.

Romans 8 applies the new creation-redemption imagery to the cosmos. This includes humanity but enlarges the scope of God's redemptive purpose to include all of creation. There, he envisions the entire creation awaiting "with eager longing" (Rom. 8:19) to "be set free from its bondage to decay" (v. 21). The picture Paul presents is that of a cosmos in the process of becoming something it now is not. It is presently "groaning in travail" (v. 22; the literal meaning is that of a woman in the pain and struggle of childbirth), but it has been given the promise of redemption, just as the people of God await the redemption of their bodies (v. 23). This, says Paul, is the hope by which we are saved (v. 24).

In summary, the biblical portrait of humanity involves several features drawn from an eschatological awareness:

1. The person is a product of a long heritage of development by which God has brought about a creature of reflective intelligence and moral awareness who may live in conscious awareness of the Creator-Redeemer;

2. The supreme expression of God's creative act is in Jesus Christ, who is thus the model, or paradigm, of true humanity;

3. The entire cosmos, including mankind, is incomplete but *in process* or on the way toward God's future;

4. The future will witness the emergence of a new humanity as much unlike us as we are unlike our earliest ancestors.

These elements are important for Christian perspectives on genetics. They provide a theological orientation or frame of reference for addressing the questions of *whether* geneticists might intervene and the type of person that might be developed through genetic engineering. One's view of the future makes considerable difference in assessing the desirability and/or moral acceptability of genetic manipulation.

The Biblical Hope and Human Action

Interest in the future is everywhere. Scientists paint scenarios based upon extrapolations from what they perceive as present trends. Futurologists mentally and statistically extend the lines of development from the past and the present into the future. The "end" or the "future" is not known, however. It can be present only on the basis of what has been or is known. At best, it only knows what is already experienced, it can only postulate a future. Further, this approach cannot take account of the unknown—the contingency factors that may enter history to alter the outcome of present trends.

Biblical eschatology proceeds with a different method. A Christian view of the future is more accurately expressed as "anticipation," or "prolepsis," according to Moltmann.[56] The background is Israel's experience of the promise of God within history that pointed to the fulfillment of the future. Their experience of partial fulfillment confirmed and became an earnest or pledge of completed fulfillment. The New Testament continues and deepens this posture of expectancy and promise. The "nearness of the kingdom" announces a reality that can now be experienced in faith and repentance (Matt. 3:2; 4:17; 10:7; Mark 1:15). The most profound expression of this hope, however, was in the cross and resurrection of Christ. Jesus' resurrection is a prolepsis, or experience in the present, of God's promise of a general "resurrection of the dead" (I Cor. 15:12–20). The church lives by that Easter faith. As Moltmann says: "It already lives from the future that has already been given in anticipatory form, and already realizes its potentialities in history to the extent in which it is no longer confined to the pattern of this world."[57]

This is of tremendous importance for Christian ethics, since images and models for thought and action are drawn from the future rather than from the past. Human action should anticipate the future action of God. Paradigms from the past are important ways to "understand eschatology historically and to grasp history eschatologically."[58]

However, care must be taken that theological eschatology not be directly translated into genetics. Theology has no direct correlation with science in the sense that categories or interests can be directly transferred. Just as a genetic code cannot constitute a theological definition of personhood, neither can the central model of Christian anthropology, Christ, constitute a working model for a scientific genotype. The Bible does not tell us what to do about genetics or even that anything must be done. The world of genetics is foreign to the writers of Scripture.

However, the Bible does supply a vision of the world and of reality, including an orientation toward the future, that is important for Christian thinking about genetics. The correlation is conceptual, not logical or technical. It is a matter of how one conceives of and intends the world and its future. For Christian thought, biblical eschatology establishes the framework for the manner in which the world is to be shaped. There is to be coherence between action and vision. What God intends for the future Christians must seek by their actions.

Moltmann has developed this theme as profoundly as any contemporary writer. His hope theology argued that eschatology is the foundation and motive for all theological thought.[59] Creation itself must be understood eschatologically, a point understood better by Irenaeus than Augustine.[60] The biblical orientation is always toward the future and the realization of God's promised kingdom.

Pierre Teilhard de Chardin spoke of that future as the Christ–omega point,[61] which is to be the fulfillment of humankind. Moltmann uses the biblical models of resurrection and the coming kingdom of God.[62] These form the central Christian expectations for the future. The eschatological kingdom bears God's promise of the "realization of justice, the humanizing of man, the socializing of humanity and peace for all creation."[63]

This orientation rejects the dogmatic pronouncements of the religions of epiphany which are based on notions of what is regarded as always and absolutely true. That static view of truth argues that reality is unchanging. Thus, the church draws its norms from the past, imposing them upon the present in rigid and dogmatic fashion and insisting that they be preserved as "givens" of God. Eschatological theology, on the other hand, argues that concepts of the present cannot be formed apart from a vision of the future.[64] Our hope is in God's future which is yet to be but toward which and into which God will lead his people.

This promised future provides a distinct perspective for human life in the world. People are not bound in a fixed place or to a static and absolute past. Rather, they are directed toward a moving future which offers the possibility of being truly human. That future is important for person as person or man as man. People are hoping creatures, for they are created for the future promised by God. That future has been proleptically experienced in Christ, who now forms the expectation of the future.

This has important meaning for a Christian understanding of the world and human actions within history. First, *it underscores the fact that the world can be molded.* History is open and not determined by forces beyond our control and thus destined for destruction. The world is a correlate of the Christian hope in the sense that it is transformable. As Wolfhart Pannenberg says, "The Christian view of love assumes that the existing world need not face destruction but can hope for salvation, but only if it is transformed."[65] Christians labor in hope; their actions are not doomed to futility. The promised future can be realized.

Second, *the Christian life-style is given direction and meaning by this vision.*[66] Paul called upon the Christians: "Let your manner of life be worthy of [or, in accordance with] the gospel of Christ" (Phil. 1:27). The Christian way of life is one of action informed by promise and committed to the future of humanity characterized by salvation, redemption, and fulfillment. The church's mission and the Christian's calling is to "seek" or pursue the kingdom of God. We are not simply to wait for the future but actively to seek it by transforming the present world. This is the call to "creative discipleship," which so relates to the kingdom of God as to be a part of that "creative expectation, [the] hope which sets about criticizing and transforming the present because it is open towards the universal future of the kingdom."[67] Christians are construction workers as well as interpreters. They are seekers after the future, striving to be in correspondence with it.

Faithful hoping rejects the temptation either to withdraw from the world into privation or to retreat into a paralyzing apocalypticism. Christians do not resign themselves to fate. They are not passive in the face of trends that threaten the future. Hope sets them free to accept the challenge presented by destructive trends they perceive in the present. God's promise against suffering and for new bodies and the absence of pain becomes a future to pursue. Those who share this vision can no longer simply accept reality as it comes to them. They begin to work for the redemption-transfiguration of all that creates destructive suffering.

A third factor which this vision provides is *a norm by which to test all current trends* toward the future. Whatever contradicts or stands in opposition to what God intends for the future is to be resisted.[68] A passive acceptance of "whatever happens" is a sinful and irresponsible attitude toward the world. Passivity is a denial of the Christian faith, for it is a loss of hope in God's future. It is not a matter of hoping on "in faith" when all hope is gone.[69] This is despair playing the waiting game. It is wishful thinking—hoping that God will work it out for the well-being of all, in spite of what people do with their genetic load or procreative responsibilities.

Sin is both striving to displace God and failing to work with God for a better world future. This is hopelessness, resignation, and despair, which is the ultimate sin.[70] Fearing to take hold of the wheel of history, people become victims of the inexorable forces of history. These "fearful" ones were listed first by the writers of the Apocalypse as among those whose future is eternal death (Rev. 21:8). "Perfect love casts out fear" (I John 4:18) which immobilizes and finally destroys. Christian hope is a passion for the possible, and thus refuses to accept this world as it is, for it is not the promised kingdom of God.

Finally, *motive or impetus for action is provided by the fact that human action may contribute to God's future.* People act in hope expecting and having been promised that beyond their own weakness, blindness, and self-contradiction God will use their actions in fashioning his kingdom. The future does not happen without them, but they do not shape it by themselves. "The kingdom is God's kingdom but we must seek it," says Moltmann.[71]

By this vision, people see themselves as conscious participants in the great enterprise of seeking and pursuing the future. They are caught up into the very history of God.[72] Their actions have a transcendent meaning which provides fulfillment and excitement for human life. This is a cosmic enterprise. Those who are actively engaged will participate in its outcome; those who resist or actively oppose will fail to realize the inheritance promised all those who pursue the kingdom of God. As Teilhard put it, "We have become aware that, in the great game that is being played, we are the players as well as the cards and the stakes."[73]

CHRISTIAN HOPE AND GENETIC HEALTH

Here, then, is a vision of the future that seems to provide legitimation for Christian support for efforts to pursue a future characterized by genetic health. This shared hope provides an inner consent to seek a future in which all of humanity will share the promise of God for healthier minds and stronger bodies. That future of strength and salvation grounds and legitimates our actions, decisions, thoughts, and goals. Without ever saying so, biblical eschatology gives both support and direction for genetically modifying the human race.

Sin and the Genetic Future

The first impulse for that action is in *the contradiction of God's promised future posed by genetic deterioration.* The Christian vision is that of a future in which there will be stronger bodies and minds. Genetic trends are toward decay and widespread helplessness. People have rendered an unfaithful stewardship of their procreative powers, for they have unwittingly created a future the prospects of which are bleak indeed. Humankind can be as surely destroyed by genetic weakness as by a nuclear fireball. The picture of the present must be taken with radical seriousness, for it portends a future to be avoided. Christians can neither hope for nor passively await the genetic twilight in which humanity has ceased to be human.

People have failed the plan of God not so much in their refusal to be believers but in their refusal to act in hope. Created as hopers, we have translated our vision of the future into wishful thinking or optimistic superstitition. Rather than take responsibility for the future that we seek or create, we lapse into a posture of "waiting for God" to act to redeem us from our own malaise.

The genetic crisis of the present is therefore a crisis of faith *and* of hope. It is a crisis that symbolizes human sin in a dramatic and ultimate way. People have contributed the primary ingredients in genetic decay. By failing to exercise constraint in the use of procreative powers; by refusing to accept responsibility for the genetic health of offspring; by tolerating and even encouraging environmental factors that contribute to genetic mutations and by resisting efforts to discover correctives, we have fallen short of "the glory [revelation] of God" (Rom. 3:23).

Genetic Ills and the Wrath of God. To the extent that genetic ills can be traced to human irresponsibility such suffering may also be regarded as the wrath of God. According to the apostle Paul, "The wrath of God is revealed from heaven against all ungodliness and wickedness of men who by their wickedness suppress the truth" (Rom. 1:18). God is related to history and nature as Judge as well as Creator and Redeemer. His righteous will judges the rebellious acts of humanity and brings them to account. God's wrath is experienced as the consequences of sin. Defying or denying the will of God does not go unpunished. God gives us up (Rom. 1:24–26, 28) to the suffering which will inevitably attend defiance of his will.

This does not mean that all such actions have been willfully or knowingly in opposition to God's will. Many such actions have been altruistic. At other times ignorance has been at fault, as in the impact of drugs that produce genetic damage. They were marketed in ignorance of their consequences. Even so, sin is involved. In failing to will genetic health and carefully screen against those factors that do damage, we have acted irresponsibly and now suffer the consequences.

Genetic Deformity and the Providence of God. Not all deformities are the consequences of human negligence, of course. Many genetic ills are the consequence of random mutations. Nature is constantly changing and those changes are frequently in our genes. This poses the problem of the providence of God.

Some people argue that all genetic handicaps are the result of the direct action of God. C. Everett Koop explains infant deformity in this way. He says that God's speech to Moses answers the question: "Who has made man's mouth? Who makes him dumb, or deaf, or seeing, or blind? Is it not I, the LORD?" (Ex. 4:11).[74] Usually the explanation insists that God has sent such suffering to punish someone for the person's sin. This interpretation of God's statement to Moses is highly questionable. The context was Moses' reluctance to become God's spokesman, fearing he would not be persuasive. "Dumb," "deaf," and "blind" are metaphors of speaking and understanding God's truth. Plainly, this passage has nothing to do with genetic deformity. Using Scripture in this manner not only poses the issue of right exegesis but the far more significant question of the moral nature of God. Jesus emphatically and explicitly rejected such explanations (see Matt. 12:22–36; Luke 11:14–23).

Where genetic illness is not traceable to human sin, people are confronted with the problem of evil in the natural process. For this dilemma, there is no easy or entirely satisfactory answer. However, two things can be affirmed. First, God does not *cause* such things to happen. The Christian understanding of God is that he is love (I John 4:8) and that his actions are good (Matt. 19:17). The basis and framework of all Christian statements about God are established by these perspectives.

In the tradition of dualism, the explanation for natural evil is found in Satan, or the evil one. The Book of Job explains Job's suffering as the adversary's (Satan's) way of testing Job. This is an important step in theodicy in that God is not directly but only *indirectly* to blame for what happened to Job. God *permitted* one of his own entourage to cause Job's pain (Job 1:6ff.)

Martin Luther declared that radical fetal deformity was caused by Satan. He said that "monster babies" were made by the devil, not by God.[75] While such a theodicy poses as many problems as it resolves, it has the virtue of refusing to attribute such actions to God. Luther plainly saw that infant deformity is a sign of evil, not of divine providence. Christians with a biblical understanding of evil will avoid resorting to pious rhetoric searching for the "hidden" or "mysterious" purposes of God for explanations for such experiences. Shakespeare put it strongly:

> 'Tis too much prov'd—that with devotion's visage
> And pious action, we do sugar o'er
> The devil himself.
>
>   *(Hamlet* 3.1.47)

The second thing to note is that natural evil confronts us with the problem of an unfinished universe. The natural order is not perfect in the sense of working properly or for the benefit of God's creatures every time. Science reminds us of the randomness and chance at work in the creative process. In every conception there are literally billions of possibilities in the genetic code that might take place. Any alteration in a single gene may result in illness or deformity. The truly amazing thing is that the process works with such harmony as it does. The biblical portrait of God's creative work is one of process and change. God begins with chaos and brings order by "brooding over" or moving within the process. The entire cosmos is a vast movement or process in time from both theological and scientific perspectives.

Evil is therefore a part of the unfinished aspect of the universe. Not every aspect of pain and suffering is the consequence of sinful acts on the part of people. Certainly some genetic problems are, as the thalidomide experience shows. We also know that pathogens in our environment are probably the primary cause of cancer and certainly contribute to genetic deformity, as the tragedy of the Love Canal demonstrates. But most genetic deformities are not the direct result of human sin (John 9:3). The evil ingredient in the process itself creates a tension with the divine plan for the redemption of the cosmos. Paul portrayed the travail of the universe in Romans 8. Tornadoes, tidal waves, hurricanes, and volcanic eruptions have their counterpart in genetic deformities in the human species. All are part of the processes of nature and point to the unfinished and dynamic aspects of creation.

Divine Providence and Human Stewardship. God calls people to participate with him to control and work against the injurious elements in nature. Paul declared that "in everything, as we know, [the Spirit] co-operates for good with those who love God and are called according to his purpose" (Rom. 8:28, NEB). The promise is that God is working along with us to bring about that which is good. This requires an ethic of choice, not chance. People are not to be passive victims of chance but active participants in seeking the health of our offspring. On the genetic front that will require not only attempting to remove or correct harmful genetic features but making those tragic but heroic choices concerning the termination of a pregnancy when it is known that the fetus is radically deformed. Because of the intricate but direct relation of genes to behavior that is moral, this could be extended to include warrants for terminating those pregnancies resulting from rape. Abortion under such circumstances is not working against God but with him.

Those who want doctors to always "keep alive" but never "take life" have a contradictory posture toward science. They see the problem of evil in human suffering but want only to deal with consequences or end results. It is "forbidden territory" to deal with genetic problems at their source. Though they argue that nature's way is God's way, they also want doctors to intervene to prevent spontaneous miscarriages even when the fetus is terribly malformed. They cannot have it both ways. To adopt the passive, noninterventionist approach is to undermine religious support for medical science at every level.

A more consistent clue is found in the notion of Christian stewardship. People are workers with God, seeking to bring about the good of the entire created order—in people and nature alike. Our knowledge of the processes that help or hinder give us a divine mandate to make choices that help rather than hinder. God wills that choices be made so that chance does not have dominion. We may make decisions to abort as stewards of genetic knowledge and as guardians of the future.

Hope and Planning

The second impulse for genetic action is found in *the requirement for planning for the future.* What is hoped for must be planned as an "anticipatory disposition toward the future."[76] The more the human condition is affected, the more important it is to plan for change in a desirable direction. Eschatological hope is neither blind nor irrational. It requires and receives direction both by the God of the future and by those who pursue that vision. The promised kingdom has content, it is not a vacuous and empty hunch or wishful thinking. Knowing something of the future requires intelligent planning and thoughtful pursuit of the goals being sought, the directions being followed, or the new creation being fashioned. The "seekers of the kingdom" are not blindly to grope for the future but intelligently, diligently, and persistently plan their path. The task is to propel history toward specific goals.

Hopeful enthusiasm may be nothing more than misguided optimism. The vision of the future must not sever the nerve of deliberation and reflective strategizing. The complexity of the issues as well as the ambiguities of choice must be taken into account.

Planning is also related to the nature of human personality. With the advent of humanity, reflective thought has replaced instinct. Evolution has become conscious of itself. With consciousness, the human being has developed the ability to exercise responsible management of the individual as reflective substance. Knowledge of is responsibility for.

This special attribute of what it means to be human underscores humanity's moral responsibility for the future. To leave the future to chance is the path to extinction and destruction.[77] Passivity denies the very being of the individual, while planning asserts the uniqueness of humanity.

The threat of genetic decay challenges us to prevent that catastrophe. Our response to the genetic dilemma will test the fabric of the human resolve to develop curative techniques to prevent decay and assure longevity for the human species. This is also a test of faith—a living response to the God who invites our participation in his work toward the future of his creation. Only a propositional notion of faith insists on preserving structures that are deteriorating. Faith as responsive hope is a pilgrimage from the city of death and decay to the land of strength and life. It is not a matter of waiting for "God to kill us all in the end,"[78] but of working with God toward "the redemption of our bodies" (Rom. 8:23) and the gift of life.

This requires *a morality of means* that is suited for planning the human genetic future. "Reflective substance requires reflective treatment," as Teilhard said. Noting the contrast between the vast numbers of human beings who are "misshapen subjects" and animal societies with flawless members, he declared that thought needs to be given to the medical and moral factors that are needed to replace the crude forces of natural selection if genetic deterioration is to be suppressed. Rather than random development, what is needed for the future of humanity is a nobly human form of eugenics, on "a standard worthy of our personalities."[79] The ultimate goal is not just to ameliorate the ills of patients but to start people off with healthy genes.[80]

Preventing birth defects is more desirable than either managing their symptoms (euphenics) or eliminating the most seriously damaged through genetic abortion or neonatal infanticide. These are measures unworthy of our personalities. At the present level of human knowledge (ignorance), however, we are confronted with tragic and undesirable alternatives. Aborting for genetic reasons may be necessary. But it is only a penultimate action offering no "solution" to the genetic crisis even if practiced on a wide scale.

What is needed is the perfection of techniques to prevent genetic anomalies. Pediatric surgeon C. Everett Koop, however, wants to prohibit all abortions *and* terminate all genetic research![81] That is to will the premature death and extensive deformity from handicap or illness of countless unborn generations. The morality of correcting genetic ills must be set against the morality of condemning the human race to genetic death. Unless and until we are willing to say that God intends genetic deformities and the decay of the human race we cannot and should not say that genetic engineering is opposed to his will. Only people can develop strategies that are needed to correct difficulties that are perceived and understood. When these techniques are used to bless and not curse the human race and to assure a more noble future, they are moral in nature.

Genetic Utopia and Christian Hope

The Christian hope for the future should not be confused with the evolutionary optimism that undergirds the utopian vision of some geneticists. The "promise" of genetic engineering is often heard as nothing less than a golden age of bliss and immortality. Science is portrayed as the salvation of humankind. The future hope thus offered is that of a world free of viral or bacterial infections; the eradication of pain and suffering both by eliminating pain-producing agents and by developing psychopharmacological means to control one's state of mind; personal immortality made possible by replaceable parts and control over the aging process; and, finally, superior intelligence, strength, and social graces to be enjoyed by everyone. In short, we are promised a world of *Homo superior.*

Reinhold Niebuhr has shown how the utopian vision has frequently employed Christian theological conceptions. The goals of the Christian future become the promises of grandiose science. These represent a combination of confidence in human reason, a high view of human nature, the conquest of nature, and social progress. To these are added a type of benevolent providence that guides the entire process toward the Golden Age. The providential power may be construed as the Christian God, evolution, or historical currents.[82]

Christian eschatology, however, is an optimism with regard to the promised kingdom of God, not the promises of technological wizardry. The Christian hope gives encouragement and direction for human effort to combat evil, but it is not a promise that technology can or will accomplish what God alone can do. The future that is technically possible is not to be identified with the hoped-for kingdom of God.[83] God's kingdom always stands against the accomplishments of the world in transcendence and judgment.

The biblical understanding of the nature of the universe itself qualifies the human dream and adds realism to utopian dreams. Christian eschatological expectations include the dimension of struggle against evil until the end. Whatever future science may accomplish will be tinged with sin and difficulty. Perfection belongs only to God; it is not a human possibility. Christians recognize the limitations under which they labor.

The story of the Fall is a reminder of the conditions under which all human striving takes place. Evil attends the very processes of nature and creation, and infects and affects all human striving. From the beginning human freedom is seen in respect to the choices that must be made between good and evil. Ambiguity belongs to reality. Mixed results can therefore be expected even from those actions prompted by the best of motives and the most noble of visions. Every solution creates an attendant problem. The hopes that enliven blueprints for action seem always to have a catch—a disappointing, unexpected, and frustrating factor.

Leon Kass describes the dilemma by saying that we cannot maximize all the benefits of science. Several goals promoted by scientists conflict with one another, as in efforts to check population growth versus the attempt to develop techniques to enable people to have children. Genetics poses a critical problem. Extending the lives of those with genetic disease conflicts with efforts to eliminate deleterious genes from the human population.[84]

What the scientist describes as a technical dilemma, the theologian describes as a metaphysical problem. Sin and evil limit the human ability to exercise control over the forces of nature. Reducing the death rate exacerbates the population explosion; overcoming natural selection, we jeopardize our genetic well-being; destroying "harmful" pests, we create an ecological crisis; and in managing pain, we develop a drug-oriented culture. This experience in life points to the truth of the biblical understanding of human life and reality. The story of human sin is a paradigm that exposes all visions of perfection for the falsehoods they project.

The experience of Adam and Eve is recapitulated in all of us. They are truly the primeval pair—a paradigm of conscious existence torn between the expectancy of the imaginative vision and the limitations of the human possibility. Every joy is accompanied by sadness; every altruistic motive is attended by selfishness. The joy of childbirth is qualified by pain (Gen. 3:16); the excitement of child-rearing is tinged with the sorrow of sibling rivalry (Gen. 4:5); the thrill of brotherly love is marred by fratricide (Gen. 4:8); the challenge of work is accompanied by drudgery, disappointment, and pain (Gen. 3:17–19).

Every technological promise of perfection in a future utopia is unrealistic, misguided, and manipulative. It fails to take seriously the problem of evil in human experience. This lack of realism breeds despair, disillusionment, and hostility when its promises are compared with what it is able to produce. "The God of the machine who promised everything to everyone seems now like an evil spirit, who draws everything to destruction," says Moltmann.[85]

Thus, there is little question that genetic knowledge will concentrate powers in the hands of the few.[86] This can be acknowledged without withdrawing support for genetics. Medical science *already* concentrates power in the hands of a few. Poorly distributed medical resources defy the vision of medicine as the benefactor of humanity. It benefits *some* people, especially those wealthy enough to purchase its goods and services. We can also reasonably predict that harmful agents will be artificially produced and that chimeras will be produced. We can also know with reasonable certainty that not all will benefit from genetic knowledge. The proposed cures themselves will work to the detriment of some.

These difficulties belong to the unfinished universe and human limitation. As long as human freedom has any meaning and as long as nature and history have any interaction, total control by human beings will not be possible. The processes of nature may and do lend themselves to a certain degree of understanding and thus of limited intervention and control. But the task is much larger and more complex than the human mind can presently envision.

Few scientists entertain the megalomaniacal notion that all of nature can be subjected to human control. Those who do are to that degree out of touch with reality—the reality of nature and history. Sin will always attend the human enterprise, and evil will permeate the processes of nature. Mutations will arise and continue to affect human well-being. The biblical reminder/warning is that human powers are always limited. The vision of possibilities always exceeds the possibilities of action and design. Of such dreams are made our technological utopias.

"HOMO FUTURUS"

The genotype of future human beings is an area in which the interests of science and religion meet. Both are prompted by their concern for human well-being and work with a certain eschatological vision. The points of disagreement are in terms of their central models that shape the vision of reality out of which plans are developed and decisions are made.

The Crucial Issue: The Paradigm of the Human

Decisions about genetic engineering pose the critical issue of the nature of personhood and those qualities which ought to be preserved and/or programmed into people of the future. Religious support can be given for a degree of genetic control. Certainly those techniques which can prevent genetic handicap or illness are to be encouraged. The critical questions arise with the prospect of actually designing the genetic details (genotype) of future people. For Christians, the intellectual, moral, and spiritual capacities of personhood are of primary concern. Efforts will therefore focus, not on attempting to *prevent* genetic tampering, but on influencing the personal capacities of *Homo futurus.*

The Christian understanding of personhood is centered in the concept of *imago Dei.* What it means to be a human being is to possess those capacities which indicate and reflect godlikeness in human life. The features of *imago Dei* are outlined in the biblical portrait of God's creating Adam and Eve—male and female—in his image. These qualities include reflective intelligence, moral awareness, God consciousness, and relational or social capacities. From these come such abilities as imagination, self-consciousness, self-transcendence, creativity, the capacity for love, and the ability to make decisions based on moral considerations.

The aim of God's creative activity in history and nature has been to bring about personhood that is perfectly responsive to him. In Christ, that purpose has been realized (Eph. 1: 9–10). Thus, the paradigm of true personhood for the Christian is to be found in Jesus Christ. He is "truly man" and thus the norm for all thinking about what it means to be truly human.

This theological and biblical truth is important for Christian thought concerning paradigms or models of personhood for *Homo futurus.* Theology can hardly be directly translated into genetics, of course. Acknowledging Christ as "true man" does not give exact specifications for the genetic engineers. We have no knowledge of Jesus' genotype or his phenotype to serve as such a blueprint. These are beyond finding out or duplicating. Even so, Christ remains the man-of-the-future for Christian anthropology. That image will give guidance as a model for any desirable or nonexpendable traits that should characterize those who come after us. He is not a blueprint, but a paradigm—a normative model for seeking what we are to become and what we shall will others to be.

The importance of the central paradigm for personhood can hardly be exaggerated. At stake is the awareness that our genetic makeup constitutes our basic intellectual, physical, moral, and spiritual capacities. All are important in the biblical portrait. But not all scientists share this perspective. The "person" that will be programmed, however, will reflect the interests and ideas of the engineer or of those who make the design decisions. Scientists are inclined to stress the need for greater intelligence, longevity, and physical strength. These capacities, unchecked by moral and spiritual capacities, could lead to a tyranny best described as demonic. Some of the worst tyrants of history have had all these traits. Greater intelligence will also enhance the cunning and cruel ways in which the powers of evil can be exercised over others. Greater strength is not desirable for those who are sociopathic. Longevity might contribute to duration of reigns of terror. Death at times signals an abrupt change for the better in historical epochs. Moltmann has reminded us that the "Christian hope is not directed toward the 'total man,' but toward the 'new man.' "[87]

Biblically informed people will therefore press to ensure that *Homo futurus* is a moral and spiritual creature as well as a strong and intelligent one. Insofar as that is done, Christians can welcome and cooperate with efforts at genetic modification. One scientist advocated developing future people with the following characteristics: creativity, wisdom, brotherliness, loving-kindness, perceptivity, expressivity, joy of life, fortitude, vigor, and longevity.[88] That list has interesting parallels to the virtues cited for Christian cultivation in the writings of Paul (see Gal. 5:22f.; Phil. 4:8). Christians find common meeting ground and room for dialogue with such scientists.

Features of Personhood

Gabriel Fackre argues that responsibility, freedom, and futurity are indispensable to being human and nonnegotiable features of *Homo futurus*.[89] These are the traits that make it possible for people to be truly human and thus manifest *imago Dei*. Three capacities should be isolated for emphasis, however. These are faith, love, and hope (I Cor. 13: 13). While these are known as the three great theological virtues, they are also basic to Christian understandings of personhood.

Faith is the uniquely human capacity for God-consciousness and responsive obedience. Self-transcendence is most uniquely focused in the ability to relate to the transcendence at the heart of the universe. In biblical terms, this is the Creator, Sustainer, and Redeemer who is revealed supremely in the incarnation. Here, conscious existence is related to purposive and meaningful existence. Humankind did not just happen, but was created by One who wills our existence and who willingly enters into relationship with us. Faith makes true humanness possible, for it is the truest reflection of its ultimate origins and goal. Relating to transcendence also sets science in the context of worship and thus checks the tendency to become an autonomous and/or demonic force. The capacity for responsiveness in faith thus ought not to be removed from *Homo futurus.*

Love, which is the revealed norm of all human conduct (Deut. 6:5; Matt. 22:37) and the essence of God (I John 4:8), is basic to humanness. This is the power at both personal and corporate levels that constrains evil in the world. Love is necessary to our function as people and our development of ego strength and value formation. It also mitigates intergroup rivalry and provides power to create community. Little wonder it is an absolute command of God. It is a universal need of humankind. In the ability to give and receive love, our highest human capacities are realized.

Hope is the capacity for futurity. True persons are hopers living with anticipation and expectation of the future and ordering their lives accordingly. This is the ingredient in human life that resists ills and injustice in the present because people can envision a different future. Hope keeps the prisoner alive, encouraging the life of the spirit against all forms of bondage. As hopers, people can transcend the present. Thus one can live prospectively, awaiting but working toward a world that is not yet but can be. This is how people act in ways shaped by shared values and visions. Hope is the mainspring of the creative impulse and those inventions which serve to alleviate unnecessary and burdensome pain. Thus, Fackre can say that those "forms of biotechnical self-control that embody *shalom,* release from imprisonment, and enlarge the capacity for seizing the future are to be received with thanksgiving and praise."[90]

Guidelines and Constraints

Beyond these characteristics of personhood that should be non-negotiable, further principles can be cited that serve as constraints against other forms of possible abuse of genetic power.

The first is that *no one phenotype should become normative.* There is no single or superior ideal specimen or race in the human family. Racial or group ideologies of superiority should be resisted as evidences of pride and arrogance. The Bible witnesses to God as Creator and Redeemer of all people regardless of racial, sexual, or class distinctions (Gal. 3:28; Acts 17:26). Christian theology focuses on the importance of inner sources of thought and conduct, not on external appearances. Thus, genotype, or genetic patterning, is much more important than phenotype or external appearance.

Positively, this will require that genetic variety be maintained. Racial and cultural mix is still important, reflecting the variety at the core of God's creativity and the extent of the divine concern for all people. On the other hand, this is no license to create novel phenotypes out of scientific curiosity. Grotesque or highly unusual physical features create problems of self-acceptance and self-identity. It would be cruel and unloving consciously to create persons whose physical features are repulsive or highly unusual.

A second principle is that *no one genotype should be mass produced.* Individuality belongs to personhood. Mass production is depersonalizing and dehumanizing. The capacity for self-awareness is the ability to say "I" with awareness of difference and uniqueness. Similarity is requisite for community, but selfhood is contradicted by sameness. The integrity of the individual is therefore to be preserved. Everyone should be a unique one.

A third principle is that *political control of genetic science is to be resisted.* While the public frequently turns to government to control by regulation the perceived "dangers" of scientific experimentation, the graver risk is that government will use science for its own purposes. The Nazi horror is a reminder of the evils created by scientific technology controlled by totalitarian politics. The Christian account of evil recognizes that its most demonic form is political ideology and tyranny. The beast of Revelation 13 is a constant reminder that political power may be used for demonic designs. Science must not become the servant of political ideology. Its reason for being in the Christian perspective is that of aiding human well-being for the glory of God (Matt. 9:8).

A final principle is that *personal freedom is to be enhanced,* not limited by prenatal programming. The person's ability to live as a free moral agent who is able to make choices is here the concern. Freedom in the biblical context is not freedom to do anything, but to do the will of God. Freedom is to live according to God's intention that every person be truly human. Those genetic arrangements which condemn people never to know what it means to make decisions live in a subhuman bondage. Science should attempt to make it possible for every child to develop the awareness of being human. Further, genetic factors now place behavioral burdens on countless people. These may contribute to compulsive and destructive behavior and these should be of concern to geneticists. When and if it is clearly demonstrated that chromosomal arrangements pattern a tendency to violent or anti-social behavior, correcting this genetic feature would be mandated by good morals. Not only would society benefit but the individual would be liberated from a terrible bondage. The principle is that any genetic linkage to compulsive behavior that is destructive to the self and/or society ought to be corrected. That will help to assure human freedom and social health.

Conclusion

The genetic crisis of our day poses the dilemma of human stewardship in a unique but unavoidable way. The apocalyptic fears of geneticists provide a point of dialogue with Christian eschatology. In this area, as in other biblical issues, the Bible does not give us clear answers as to what should or should not be done. But it does provide definite guidance in terms of its understanding of reality and its paradigms for the future. Clearly there is no knowledge that is religiously "off limits," but true knowledge is an awareness that there are many things and goals beyond our limits. False promises are as dangerous as deliberate deception, for they substitute illusion for reality and seek a kingdom that is neither promised nor possible by human action alone. The end is disillusionment and despair, the bitter but predictable legacies of the perpetrators of the false vision.

Biblical eschatology does seem to provide warrant for genetic studies and certain forms of genetic manipulation. As stewards of the powers that belong to reflective intelligence and as bearers of the image of God we are called to avoid death by genetic deterioration and fashion strong bodies and genuinely moral capacities that enable humankind more perfectly to bear the image of God.

NOTES

Chapter 1. BIOETHICS: SCIENCE AND HUMAN VALUES

1. Christiaan Barnard, *Good Life Good Death: A Doctor's Case for Euthanasia and Suicide* (Prentice-Hall, 1980).

2. *Courier-Journal* (Louisville, Ky.), March 3, 1978, p. A-8.

3. *Diamond* v. *Chakrabarty,* June 16, 1980.

4. Jacques Ellul, *The Technological Society,* trans. John Wilkinson (Vintage Books, 1964), pp. 135ff.; also Jacques Ellul, *To Will and to Do,* trans. C. Edward Hopkin (Pilgrim Press, 1969), Ch. 11, "Technological Morality."

5. Herman J. Muller, "The Guidance of Human Evolution," *American Naturalist,* Vol. 100 (1966), p. 519.

6. Caryl Rivers, "Grave New World," *Saturday Review,* April 8, 1972, pp. 23–27.

7. Alvin Toffler, *Future Shock* (Random House, 1970).

8. Van R. Potter, *Bioethics: Bridge to the Future* (Prentice-Hall, 1971), p. 82.

9. Emil Brunner, *The Divine Imperative,* trans. Olive Wyon (Westminster Press, 1947), p. 86.

10. See Potter, *Bioethics: Bridge to the Future,* p. 2.

11. Clayton L. Thomas (ed.), *Taber's Cyclopedic Medical Dictionary* (F. A. Davis Co., 1970), p. E-64.

12. Willard Gaylin, "Foreword," in *Moral Problems in Medicine,* ed. Samuel Gorowitz et al. (Prentice-Hall, 1976), p. xvi.

13. Paul Ramsey, *The Patient as Person* (Yale University Press, 1970).

14. Eliot Friedson, *Profession of Medicine: A Study of the Sociology of Applied Knowledge* (Dodd, Mead & Co., 1970), p. 208.

15. Warren T. Reich (ed.), *Encyclopedia of Bioethics* (Free Press, 1978), p. xix.

16. See Sidney Callahan, "Bioethics as a Discipline," *Hastings Center Studies*, Vol. 1, No. 1 (1973), p. 71.

17. Edward O. Wilson, *On Human Nature* (Harvard University Press, 1978), p. 1.

18. Alfred N. Whitehead, *Science and the Modern World* (Free Press, 1953), p. 181.

Chapter 2. THE BIBLE AND BIOETHICAL DECISION-MAKING

1. Leander Keck, *Taking the Bible Seriously* (Association Press, 1962), p. 123.

2. Thomas B. Maston, *Biblical Ethics* (World Publishing Co., 1967).

3. Johannes Hempel, "Ethics in the Old Testament," in *The Interpreter's Dictionary of the Bible,* ed. George A. Buttrick et al. (Abingdon Press, 1962), Vol. 2, pp. 153–161.

4. Kornelis Miskotte, *When the Gods Are Silent,* trans. John W. Doberstein (Harper & Row, 1967).

5. As in Jack T. Sanders, *Ethics in the New Testament* (Fortress Press, 1975).

6. See James L. Houlden, *Ethics and the New Testament* (Penguin Books, 1973), and Victor Paul Furnish, *Theology and Ethics in Paul* (Abingdon Press, 1968).

7. James M. Gustafson, *Theology and Christian Ethics* (United Church Press, 1974), p. 122.

8. David H. Kelsey, *The Uses of Scripture in Recent Theology* (Fortress Press, 1975), pp. 152–153.

9. Brevard S. Childs, *Biblical Theology in Crisis* (Westminster Press, 1970), p. 131.

10. Keck, *Taking the Bible Seriously,* p. 126.

11. Bruce C. Birch and Larry L. Rasmussen, *Bible and Ethics in the Christian Life* (Augsburg Publishing House, 1976), p. 144.

12. Kelsey, *The Uses of Scripture in Recent Theology,* p. 153.

13. Henry D. Aiken, *Reason and Conduct* (Alfred A. Knopf, 1962), pp. 67 and 68f.

14. See Glen H. Stassen, "Critical Variables in Christian Social Ethics," in *Issues in Christian Ethics,* ed. Paul D. Simmons (Broadman Press, 1980), p. 57.

15. James M. Gustafson, *Christian Ethics and the Community,* ed. Charles M. Sweazey (Pilgrim Press, 1971), p. 102.

16. Ibid., p. 118.

17. Stassen, "Critical Variables in Christian Social Ethics," in Sim-

mons (ed.), *Issues in Christian Ethics,* p. 57. See also his article in *Journal of Religious Ethics,* Spring 1977, pp. 9–37.

18. Edward L. Long, Jr., "The Use of the Bible in Christian Ethics," *Interpretation,* Vol. 19, No. 2 (April 1965), p. 149.

19. H. E. Everding and Dana Wilbanks, *Decision Making and the Bible* (Judson Press, 1975), p. 24.

20. Stassen, "Critical Variables in Christian Social Ethics," in Simmons (ed.), *Issues in Christian Ethics,* p. 57.

21. John C. Murray, *Principles of Conduct* (London: Tyndale Press, 1957), p. 24.

22. "The Chicago Statement on Biblical Inerrancy" (Oakland, Calif.), Art. V.

23. Ibid., Arts. VI and VIII.

24. Murray, p. 154.

25. Edward L. Long, Jr., *A Survey of Christian Ethics* (Oxford University Press, 1967), p. 45.

26. See Henlee H. Barnette, *Introducing Christian Ethics* (Broadman Press, 1954), p. 8.

27. Andrew R. Osborne, *Christian Ethics,* quoted by Long, "The Use of the Bible in Christian Ethics," p. 155.

28. Albert Knudson, *The Principles of Christian Ethics* (Abingdon Press, 1943), p. 39.

29. Barnette, *Introducing Christian Ethics,* pp. 19f.

30. Ibid., p. 23.

31. Ibid.

32. Henlee H. Barnette, *The Church and the Ecological Crisis* (Wm. B. Eerdmans Publishing Co., 1972).

33. Arthur Dyck, *On Human Care: An Introduction to Ethics* (Abingdon Press, 1977).

34. Long, *A Survey of Christian Ethics,* p. 117.

35. Everding and Wilbanks, *Decision-Making and the Bible,* p. 31.

36. Paul Lehmann, *Ethics in a Christian Context* (Harper & Row, 1963), p. 348.

37. Joseph Fletcher, *Situation Ethics: The New Morality* (Westminster Press, 1966), p. 49.

38. Leonard Hodgson et al., *On the Authority of the Bible* (London: S.P.C.K., 1960), p. 8.

39. I am using "Christian" in a descriptive sense to indicate those actions which correspond to one's commitment to Christ. This is a different meaning from that used by Kelsey. See above at note 12.

40. See James M. Gustafson, *Christ and the Moral Life* (Harper & Row, 1968), who outlines five models.

41. Fundamentalism may take exception to this, for it places such

a stress on divinity that Jesus is effectively removed from the processes of moral decision-making that people confront. What was important about Jesus was his atoning work, not his teachings. See Georgia Harkness, *John Calvin: The Man and His Ethics* (Abingdon Press, 1958), p. 72.

42. H. Richard Niebuhr, *Christ and Culture* (Harper & Brothers, 1951), p. 11.

43. Everding and Wilbanks, *Decision-Making and the Bible*, p. 25. This is not a serious or scholarly approach to the Bible, but it occurs frequently in religious discussions and thus merits attention.

44. John H. Yoder, *The Politics of Jesus* (Wm. B. Eerdmans Publishing Co., 1972). Yoder argues that Jesus' hermeneutic was humanitarian concern. Thus, Jesus could call on the Jews to observe Jubilee as required under Old Testament Law while violating ceremonial requirements when they did not serve human need.

45. Brunner, *The Divine Imperative*, pp. 132, 134.

46. Milton L. Rudnick, *Christian Ethics for Today: An Evangelical Approach* (Baker Book House, 1979), p. 94.

47. Lehmann, *Ethics in a Christian Context*, p. 85.

48. See James M. Gustafson, *Can Ethics Be Christian?* (University of Chicago Press, 1975), p. 26.

49. H. Richard Niebuhr, *Radical Monotheism and Western Culture* (University of Nebraska Press, 1960), pp. 11–18.

50. Brunner, *The Divine Imperative*, p. 138.

51. Gustafson, *Can Ethics Be Christian?* pp. 73–75.

52. Ernest Becker, *The Denial of Death* (Free Press, 1973), p. 278.

53. See H. Page Lee, "Methodology in Christian Ethics," in Simmons (ed.), *Issues in Christian Ethics*, p. 49, and Stassen, in ibid., pp. 62f.

54. Gustafson, *Theology and Christian Ethics*, p. 141.

55. See Edward O. Wilson, *Sociobiology: The New Synthesis* (Harvard University Press, 1975), p. 547, who says that anatomical differences account for the distinctively human.

Chapter 3: ABORTION: THE BIBLICAL AND HUMAN ISSUES

1. Francis Schaeffer and C. Everett Koop, *Whatever Happened to the Human Race?* (Fleming H. Revell Co., 1979), p. 23.

2. For historical summaries, see David R. Mace, *Abortion: The Agonizing Decision* (Abingdon Press, 1972), pp. 52ff.; Harmon L. Smith, *Ethics and the New Medicine* (Abingdon Press, 1970), pp. 26ff.; and John T. Noonan, Jr. (ed.), *The Morality of Abortion* (Harvard University Press, 1970), pp. 3ff.

3. Clyde T. Francisco, "Genesis," *Broadman Bible Commentary,* Vol. 1 (Broadman Press, 1973), p. 406.

4. Aristotle, *Politics* VII. xv. 1335.

5. Tertullian, *On the Resurrection of the Body* lix (59).

6. Tertullian, *De Anima.*

7. Martin Luther, *Luther's Works,* Vol. 45, ed. Walther I. Brandt (Muhlenberg Press, 1962), pp. 396–397.

8. George H. Kieffer, *Bioethics: A Textbook of Issues* (Addison-Wesley Publishing Co., 1979), p. 159.

9. *Roe* v. *Wade,* U.S. Supreme Court, Jan. 22, 1973.

10. See Kieffer, *Bioethics: A Textbook of Issues,* pp. 173–174, for a more comprehensive list.

11. See William Ray Arney and William H. Trescher, "Trends in Attitudes Toward Abortion," *Perspectives,* May/June 1977, p. 118.

12. Harold O. J. Brown, *Death Before Birth* (Thomas Nelson, 1977), p. 119. See also Donald P. Shoemaker, *Abortion, the Bible and the Christian* (Hayes Publishing Co., 1976), p. 35, and Schaeffer and Koop, *Whatever Happened to the Human Race?*

13. Cited by Richard A. McCormick, S.J., "Abortion," *America,* June 19, 1965, p. 898.

14. Karl Barth, *Church Dogmatics,* III/4, trans. A. T. Mackay et al. (Edinburgh: T. & T. Clark, 1961), p. 415.

15. John R. W. Stott, "Reverence for Human Life," *Christianity Today,* June 9, 1972, p. 10.

16. Daniel Callahan, *Abortion: Law, Choice, and Morality* (Macmillan Co., 1970), Ch. 11.

17. Paul Ramsey, "Points in Deciding About Abortion," in Noonan (ed.), *The Morality of Abortion,* pp. 66–67. See also Schaeffer and Koop, *Whatever Happened to the Human Race?* p. 41.

18. Jürgen Moltmann, "The Humanity of Living and Dying," in his *The Experiment Hope,* ed. and trans. M. Douglas Meeks (Fortress Press, 1975), p. 166.

19. Charles Hartshorne, "Ethics and the Process of Living," Conference on Religion, Ethics and the Life Process, Institute of Religion and Human Development, Texas Medical Center, March 18–19, 1979.

20. Stott, "Reverence for Human Life," p. 10.

21. Sissela Bok, "Who Shall Count as a Human Being?" in *Abortion: Pro and Con,* ed. Robert C. Perkins (Schenkman Publishing Co., 1974), p. 91.

22. See Barth, *Church Dogmatics,* III/4, pp. 327–333; and Joseph Fletcher, "Indicators of Humanhood: A Tentative Profile of Man," in *Hastings Center Report,* Vol. 2, No. 5 (1972), pp. 1–4, for a list of fifteen positive and five negative criteria or characteristics of per-

sonhood. Also see his "Four Indicators of Humanhood—The Inquiry Matures," *Hastings Center Report,* Vol. 4, No. 6 (1974), pp. 4–7.

23. Jack W. Cottrell, "Abortion and the Mosaic Law," *Christianity Today,* March 16, 1973, p. 8.

24. Bruce K. Waltke, "The Old Testament and Birth Control," *Christianity Today,* Nov. 8, 1968.

25. Brown, *Death Before Birth,* pp. 20f., esp. p. 22, where he speaks of "willful killing of innocent human beings . . . as an offense against the image of God in man."

26. See Schaeffer and Koop, *Whatever Happened to the Human Race?* pp. 85, 101. Note that Schaeffer and Koop never define "image of God." They treat it as an entity or quality that is possessed from conception.

27. Brown, *Death Before Birth,* p. 119.

28. See Paul D. Simmons, "The 'Human' as a Problem in Bioethics," *Review and Expositor,* Vol. 78, No. 1 (Winter 1981), p. 102.

29. James M. Gustafson, "A Protestant Ethical Approach," in Noonan (ed.), *The Morality of Abortion,* pp. 102ff.

30. Barth, *Church Dogmatics,* III/4, p. 418.

31. Garrett Hardin, in *Abortion and the Unwanted Child,* ed. Carl Reiterman (Springer Publishing Co., 1971), p. 5.

32. Barth, *Church Dogmatics,* III/4, p. 422.

33. Ibid.

34. Bernhard Häring, *Medical Ethics,* ed. Gabrielle L. Jean (Fides Publishers, 1973), p. 37.

35. *Courier-Journal* (Louisville, Ky.), Jan. 4, 1981, p. A-14.

36. Rabbi David Feldman, "Is Abortion Murder or Not?" *Church and Society,* Vol. 71, No. 4 (March–April 1981), p. 47.

37. Noonan (ed.), *The Morality of Abortion,* p. 9.

38. Karl Barth, *Church Dogmatics,* II/2, trans. G. W. Bromiley et al. (Edinburgh: T. & T. Clark, 1957), p. 663.

39. Barth, *Church Dogmatics,* III/4, pp. 421, 416.

40. Ibid., p. 415.

41. Ibid., p. 420.

42. See Phyllis Trible, *God and the Rhetoric of Sexuality* (Fortress Press, 1978), pp. 75–105.

43. See Edward O. Wilson, *Sociobiology: The New Synthesis,* p. 554, for a discussion of the uniqueness of human sexuality.

44. Shoemaker, *Abortion, the Bible and the Christian,* p. 30.

45. Ibid., p. 30. Shoemaker is referring to pregnancy and makes the astounding comment that this is God's testing of *men!*

46. Bruce K. Waltke, "Reflections from the Old Testament on Abortion," Presidential Address at Dec. 29, 1975, meeting of the Evangelical Theological Society, p. 11.

47. Joseph Fletcher, *Humanhood: Essays in Biomedical Ethics* (Prometheus Books, 1979), p. 138.

Chapter 4. EUTHANASIA: THE PERSON AND DEATH

1. See Elisabeth Kübler-Ross, *Questions and Answers on Death and Dying* (Macmillan Publishing Co., 1974), p. 74.
2. Bernhard Häring, *The Ethics of Manipulation* (Seabury Press, 1975), p. 106.
3. Paul Ramsey, *Fabricated Man: The Ethics of Genetic Control* (Yale University Press, 1970), p. 150 (Ramsey's italics).
4. Raymond S. Duff, "Shall These Children Live—A Conversation," *Reflection*, Vol. 72, No. 2 (Jan. 1975), p. 9.
5. Ramsey, "Points in Deciding About Abortion," in Noonan (ed.), *The Morality of Abortion*, p. 94.
6. See Paul W. Pretzel, *Understanding and Counseling the Suicidal Person* (Abingdon Press, 1972), p. 202.
7. Lael T. Wertenbaker, *Death of a Man* (Beacon Press, 1974).
8. Fletcher, *Humanhood: Essays in Biomedical Ethics*, p. 149.
9. Reinhold Niebuhr, *The Nature and Destiny of Man* (Charles Scribner's Sons, 1949), Vol. 1, p. 99.
10. Jerry B. Wilson, *Death by Decision* (Westminster Press, 1975), p. 18. Also see the brief but excellent history in Rannon Gillon, "Suicide and Voluntary Euthanasia," *Euthanasia and the Right to Death*, ed. A. B. Downing (Nash Publishing Corp., 1969), pp. 173–183. Except where otherwise indicated, the historical material in this section is drawn from these two sources.
11. See Edmond Jacob, "Death," in *The Interpreter's Dictionary of the Bible*, Vol. 1, p. 802.
12. John Donne, *Complete Poetry and Selected Prose*, ed. John Hayward (London: Nonesuch Library, 1955), pp. 420–425.
13. Albert Camus, *The Myth of Sisyphus*, trans. Justin O'Brien (Vintage Books, 1955).
14. See Stassen, "Critical Variables in Christian Social Ethics," in Simmons (ed.), *Issues in Christian Ethics*, p. 62.
15. See Gillon, "Suicide and Voluntary Euthanasia," in Downing, (ed.), *Euthanasia and the Right to Death*, p. 173.
16. See Schaeffer and Koop, *Whatever Happened to the Human Race?* p. 90, for an example of this strategy.
17. For this reason among others, Robert Veatch has suggested that it would be wise to drop the term from current discussions. See Robert M. Veatch, "Choosing Not to Prolong Death," in *Bioethics*, ed. Thomas A. Shannon (Paulist/Newman Press, 1976), p. 182.

18. Joseph Fletcher, *Morals and Medicine* (Princeton University Press, 1954), p. 172.

19. See Jacques Choron, *Suicide* (Charles Scribner's Sons, 1972), p. 97; Pretzel, *Understanding and Counseling the Suicidal Person*, p. 202; and Fletcher, *Humanhood: Essays in Biomedical Ethics*, p. 153.

20. Fletcher, *Humanhood: Essays in Biomedical Ethics*, p. 153.

21. *Courier-Journal* (Louisville, Ky.), Nov. 5, 1973.

22. Fletcher, *Humanhood: Essays in Biomedical Ethics*, p. 153.

23. Harmon Smith, *Ethics and the New Medicine*, p. 145.

24. See Karen Lebaqz, "Against the California Natural Death Act," *Hastings Center Report*, Vol. 7, No. 2 (April 1977).

25. Darrel W. Amandsen, "The Physician's Obligation to Prolong Life: A Medical Duty Without Classical Roots," *Hastings Center Report*, Vol. 8, No. 4 (Aug. 1978), pp. 23–28.

26. Fletcher, *Humanhood: Essays in Biomedical Ethics*, p. 154.

27. *Time*, Nov. 16, 1962, p. 67.

28. Fletcher, *Humanhood: Essays in Biomedical Ethics*, p. 154.

29. Ibid.

30. See Barth, *Church Dogmatics*, III/4, pp. 327–333. He lists seven features of personhood: (1) independence, (2) rationality, (3) self-awareness, (4) response-able and responsible, (5) freedom, (6) purposiveness, and (7) fellowship with others.

31. See Schaeffer and Koop, *Whatever Happened to the Human Race?*, pp. 101f.

32. William E. May, "Euthanasia, Benemortasia and the Dying," in *Moral Issues and Christian Response*, 2d ed., ed. Paul T. Jersild and Dale A. Johnson (Holt, Rinehart & Winston, 1976), p. 404.

33. See Dale Moody, *The Word of Truth* (Wm. B. Eerdmans Publishing Co., 1981), p. 487.

34. Harmon Smith, *Ethics and the New Medicine*, p. 125.

35. Paul Ramsey, "The Indignity of 'Death with Dignity,' " *Hastings Center Studies*, Vol. 2, No. 2 (May 1974), p. 56.

36. Paul Ramsey, "Death's Pedagogy," *Commonweal*, Sept. 20, 1974, p. 500.

37. Ramsey, "The Indignity of 'Death with Dignity,' " p. 56. See also Schaeffer and Koop, *Whatever Happened to the Human Race?*, p. 91.

38. *Courier-Journal* (Louisville, Ky.), March 2, 1975, p. G-7.

39. James B. Nelson, *Human Medicine* (Augsburg Publishing House, 1973), p. 129.

40. Ramsey, *The Patient as Person*, p. 63.

41. Ramsey, *Fabricated Man*, p. 99.

42. See Robert S. Morison, "Death: Process or Event?" and Leon

R. Kass, "Death as an Event: A Commentary on Robert Morison," *Science,* Aug. 20, 1971.

43. Nelson, *Human Medicine,* p. 126.

44. Harmon Smith, *Ethics and the New Medicine,* p. 165.

45. Daniel Callahan, *Abortion: Law, Choice, and Morality,* p. 387.

46. Robert M. Veatch, *Death, Dying, and the Biological Revolution* (Yale University Press, 1976), p. 42.

47. *Courier-Journal* (Louisville, Ky.), July 10, 1981, p. A-2.

48. *Courier-Journal* (Louisville, Ky.), April 14, 1978, p. D-12.

49. Ramsey, "Death's Pedagogy," p. 501.

50. See Adolf Holl, *Death and the Devil,* trans. Matthew J. O'Connell (Seabury Press, 1976), p. 118. Also see Ramsey, "Death's Pedagogy," p. 500.

51. See Alan Harrington, *The Immortalist* (Random House, 1969). See also Joel Kurtzman and Phillip Gordon, *No More Dying* (Austin, Tex.: Learning Concepts, 1976).

52. See the insightful criticism of Ernest Becker, *The Denial of Death,* pp. 266f.

53. See Reinhold Niebuhr, *The Nature and Destiny of Man,* Vol. 1, p. 174.

54. See Moody, *The Word of Truth,* p. 29, for a fuller discussion.

55. See Elisabeth Kübler-Ross, *On Death and Dying* (Macmillan Co., 1969), p. 9.

56. The story is told by G. A. Gresham, M.D., in Downing (ed.), *Euthanasia and the Right to Death,* p. 150.

57. Ramsey, *The Patient as Person,* p. 119.

58. Elisabeth Kübler-Ross, *Death: The Final Stage of Growth* (Prentice-Hall, 1975), see esp. Ch. 6.

59. Ramsey, "Death's Pedagogy," pp. 497–502.

60. See Stewart Alsop, *Stay of Execution* (J. B. Lippincott Co., 1974).

61. Ramsey, "Death's Pedagogy," p. 498.

62. Norman St. John-Stevas, "Euthanasia in England: The Growing Storm," *America,* May 2, 1970.

63. Eike-Henner W. Kluge, *The Ethics of Deliberate Death* (Kennikat Press, 1981), p. 35.

64. J. Philip Wogaman, *A Christian Method of Moral Judgment* (Westminster Press, 1977), p. 40.

65. May, "Euthanasia, Benemortasia and the Dying," in Jersild and Johnson (eds.), *Moral Issues and Christian Response,* 2d ed., p. 404.

66. John H. Yoder, "Expository Articles: Thou Shalt Not Kill—Exodus 20:13," *Interpretation,* Oct. 1980, p. 396.

67. Ramsey, *The Patient as Person*, pp. 113ff., and Dyck, *On Human Care*, p. 81.

68. See Gillon, "Suicide and Voluntary Euthanasia: Historical Perspective," in Downing (ed.), *Euthanasia and the Right to Death*, p. 190.

69. Marvin Kohl, "Understanding the Case for Beneficent Euthanasia," *Science, Medicine and Man* I:1973, pp. 111–121.

70. Dyck, *On Human Care*, p. 81.

71. Ibid., pp. 83–84.

72. Ramsey, *The Patient as Person*, p. 125.

73. The story in II Sam. 1 says the armor-bearer dispatched Saul as requested.

74. James Rachels, "Active and Passive Euthanasia," in *Ethical Issues in Death and Dying*, ed. Tom L. Beauchamp and Seymour Perlin (Prentice-Hall, 1978), pp. 240–246.

75. Quoted in *Time*, July 4, 1960, p. 38.

76. William May takes this distinction to its illogical extreme when he says that shooting a person who is trapped in a fire (which he approves) is aimed at the pain, not at the person! See May, "Euthanasia, Benemortasia and the Dying," in Jersild and Johnson (eds.), *Moral Issues and Christian Response*, 2d ed., p. 400.

77. See Glanville Williams, *The Sanctity of Life in Criminal Law* (Alfred A. Knopf, 1962), p. 288.

78. Paul Ramsey, *The Just War: Force and Political Responsibility* (Charles Scribner's Sons, 1968), p. 206.

79. Ibid., p. 406. Dyck says bluntly that "any act of taking a human life is wrong," *On Human Care*, p. 82.

80. Ramsey and others expand these two to include seven, ordinarily: (1) proper authority, (2) just cause, (3) prospect of victory; (4) last resort; (5) just intention; (6) just conduct; (7) due proportionality, i.e., good probably to be achieved must outweigh the evils that are certain to be involved.

81. Henlee H. Barnette, *Exploring Medical Ethics* (Mercer University Press, 1982), p. 130.

82. Nelson, *Human Medicine*, p. 140.

Chapter 5. THE BIBLE AND BIOTECHNICAL PARENTING

1. *The Phil Donahue Show*, dialogue with Tim Toomey, "The World's Most Unusual Father," *Family Circle*, Feb. 3, 1981.

2. Joshua Lederberg, "Foreword" to Joseph Fletcher, *The Ethics of Genetic Control* (Doubleday & Co., Anchor Press Books, 1974), p. ix at note.

3. Cited by Joe Ward in a newspaper series "The Pursuit of a Baby," 4 parts, *Courier-Journal* (Louisville, Ky.), Nov. 23, 1980, to Nov. 26, 1980.

4. See William H. Willimon, "Unto Us a Child: Personal Perspective," *Christian Century*, Dec. 19, 1979, p. 1273.

5. *Journal of the American Medical Association*, Vol. 220 (1972), p. 1356.

6. Herman J. Muller, "Genetic Progress by Voluntarily Conducted Germinal Choice," in *Moral Issues and Christian Response*, ed. Paul Jersild and Dale Johnson (Holt, Rinehart & Winston, 1971), p. 430.

7. Leon R. Kass, "New Beginnings in Life," in *The New Genetics and the Future of Man*, ed. Michael P. Hamilton (Wm. B. Eerdmans Publishing Co., 1972), p. 42.

8. See James D. Watson, "Moving Toward the Clonal Man," *Atlantic*, May 1971, p. 52.

9. See David Rorvik, *In His Image: The Cloning of a Man* (Pocket Books, 1978).

10. Toffler, *Future Shock*, pp. 215f.

11. See Häring, *Medical Ethics*, p. 92.

12. Ibid., p. 93.

13. Toffler, *Future Shock*, p. 213.

14. Ellul, *The Technological Society*, p. 143.

15. Lori B. Andrews, "Embryo Technology," *Parents*, May 1981, p. 67.

16. "Hiring Mothers," *Time*, June 5, 1978, p. 59.

17. *Courier-Journal* (Louisville, Ky.), Sept. 6, 1981, p. A-8.

18. *Doe* v. *Kelley*, quoted by George J. Annas, "Contracts to Bear a Child: Compassion or Commercialism?" *Hastings Center Report*, Vol. 11, No. 2 (April 1981), p. 23.

19. Annas, "Contracts to Bear a Child," p. 24.

20. Cited by Andrews, "Embryo Technology," p. 66.

21. Moltmann, *The Experiment Hope*, p. 166.

22. Rachel R. Smith, "Pregnancy and Childbirth as a Theological Event," *Christian Century*, Dec. 19, 1979, p. 1264.

23. Shoemaker, *Abortion, the Bible and the Christian*, p. 37.

24. Häring, *Medical Ethics*, p. 94.

25. Paul Ramsey, "Shall We Reproduce?" II, *Journal of the American Medical Association*, June 12, 1972, p. 1481.

26. Jack W. Moore, "Human In-Vitro Fertilization," *Christian Century*, April 21, 1981, p. 445.

27. See Rachel Smith, "Pregnancy and Childbirth as a Theological Event," p. 1264, who relates this particularly to the woman's relation to the child.

28. *Courier-Journal* (Louisville, Ky.), April 8, 1981, p. C-4.

29. Richard A. McCormick, *How Brave a New World?* (Double-day & Co., 1981), p. 303.

30. Barth, *Church Dogmatics,* III/4, p. 266.

31. See Ramsey, "Shall We Reproduce?" II, p. 1485.

32. *Courier-Journal* (Louisville, Ky.), May 21, 1981, p. C-1.

33. Ramsey, "Shall We Reproduce?" II, p. 1481.

34. Joseph Fletcher, "Ethical Aspects of Genetic Control," *New England Journal of Medicine,* Vol. 285 (1971), p. 776–783.

35. Joseph Fletcher, *The Ethics of Genetic Control,* p. 35.

36. Fletcher, "Ethical Aspects of Genetic Control," p. 781.

37. See McCormick, *How Brave a New World?,* p. 285.

38. Ramsey, "Shall We Reproduce?" II, p. 1481.

Chapter 6. GENETICS, THE BIBLE, AND THE HUMAN FUTURE

1. *Courier-Journal* (Louisville, Ky.), Jan. 10, 1982, p. B-4.

2. *Louisville (Ky.) Times,* March 17, 1979, p. A-10.

3. See Gerald J. Stine, *Biosocial Genetics* (Macmillan Co., 1977), and Peter Volpe, *Human Heredity and Birth Defects* (Bobbs-Merrill Co., 1971).

4. "Clue to Origins of Some Cancers Discovered," *Courier-Journal* (Louisville, Ky.), Sept. 13, 1979, p. A-8.

5. *Courier-Journal* (Louisville, Ky.), Jan. 5, 1979, p. B-4.

6. See Zsolt Harsanyi and Richard Hutton, *Genetic Prophecy: Beyond the Double Helix* (Rawson, Wade Publishers, 1981), pp. 14f.

7. *Courier-Journal* (Louisville, Ky.), July 12, 1981, pp. D-1, 4.

8. David G. Lygre, *Life Manipulation* (Walker & Co., 1979), p. 50.

9. Kieffer, *Bioethics: A Textbook of Issues,* p. 133. The term designates certain diseases that are debilitating, contagious and/or can be spread to other people through contact, e.g., TB.

10. See Stine, *Biosocial Genetics,* and Volpe, *Human Heredity and Birth Defects.*

11. Schaeffer and Koop, *Whatever Happened to the Human Race?,* pp. 71–72.

12. Cited by Thomas P. Carney, *Instant Evolution* (University of Notre Dame Press, 1980), p. 50.

13. Cited by Fletcher, *The Ethics of Genetic Control,* p. 49.

14. F. Osborn, "The Protection and Improvement of Man's Genetic Inheritance," in *The Population Crisis and the Use of World Resources,* ed. Stuart Mudd et al. (The Hague: Uitgeverij W. Junk, 1964), pp. 306–313.

15. Fletcher, *The Ethics of Genetic Control*, p. 50.

16. Ramsey, *Fabricated Man*, p. 118.

17. Kieffer, *Bioethics: A Textbook of Issues*, p. 195.

18. *Courier-Journal* (Louisville, Ky.), Feb. 23, 1980, p. A-2.

19. See Kieffer, *Bioethics: A Textbook of Issues*, p. 199, and the Ralph Nader Research Group Report, *Surgical Sterilization: Present Abuses and Proposed Regulations*. See also Patricia Donovan, "Sterilizing the Poor and Incompetent," *Hastings Center Report*, Vol. 6, No. 5 (1976), pp. 7–8.

20. Muller, "Genetic Progress by Voluntarily Conducted Germinal Choice," in Jersild and Johnson (eds.), *Moral Issues and Christian Response*, p. 430.

21. Ibid.

22. Carney, *Instant Evolution*, p. 41.

23. Ramsey, *Fabricated Man*, p. 19.

24. "Spliced Genes Used on Human Patients," *The New York Times*, Thurs., Oct. 8, 1980, p. A-31. See also Karen E. Mercola and Martin B. Cline, "The Potentials of Inserting New Genetic Information," *New England Journal of Medicine*, Nov. 27, 1980, pp. 1297–1300.

25. "Colleagues Call Genetic-Experiment of Dr. Cline Irresponsible," *Courier-Journal* (Louisville, Ky.), Nov. 9, 1980, p. G-7.

26. Fletcher, *The Ethics of Genetic Control*, p. xv.

27. Rivers, "Grave New World," *Saturday Review*, April 8, 1972, pp. 23–27.

28. Jürgen Moltmann, *Man*, trans. John Sturdy (Fortress Press, 1974), p. x.

29. Ramsey, *Fabricated Man*, p. 7.

30. C. S. Lewis, *The Abolition of Man* (Macmillan Co., 1965), pp. 46f.

31. John R. Batt, "Hippocrates as 'Big Brother': An Essay on Orwellian Medicine," in *Should Doctors Play God?* ed. Claude Frazier (Broadman Press, 1971), p. 133.

32. Lewis, *The Abolition of Man*, p. 49.

33. Moltmann, *Man*, p. 25.

34. Lewis, *The Abolition of Man*, p. 41.

35. Ibid., p. 35.

36. See Robert L. Sinsheimer, *Daedalus*, Vol. 107, No. 2 (Spring 1978), pp. 23–25.

37. Dr. Kurt Semm, quoted by Lori B. Andrews in "Embryo Technology," *Parents*, May 1981, p. 63.

38. Henry Stobb, "Christian Ethics and Scientific Control," in *The Scientist and Ethical Decisions*, ed. Charles Hatfield (Inter-Varsity Press, 1973), p. 20.

39. Paul Ramsey, "Shall We 'Reproduce'? I. The Medical Ethics of In-Vitro Fertilization," *Journal of the American Medical Association,* June 5, 1972, p. 1347.

40. In a symposium on recombinant DNA research at Princeton University, Spring, 1977. See also Ramsey, *Fabricated Man,* p. 134.

41. Samuel E. Stumpf, "Genetics and the Control of Human Development," in *A Matter of Life and Death,* ed. Harry H. Hollis, Jr. (Broadman Press, 1977), p. 115.

42. For a fuller development of the Augustinian theology, see John Hick, *Evil and the God of Love,* rev. ed. (Harper & Row, 1966), pp. 18f.

43. See Donald Johanson and Maitland Edey, *Lucy: The Beginnings of Humankind* (Simon & Schuster, 1981).

44. Theodosius Dobzhansky, "Man and Natural Selection," *American Scientist,* Vol. 49 (1961), pp. 285–299.

45. Jacques Ellul, *The Meaning of the City,* trans. Dennis Pardee (Wm. B. Eerdmans Publishing Co., 1970), p. 195.

46. Herman J. Muller, "The Guidance of Human Evolution," in *Perspectives in Biology and Medicine* (University of Chicago Press, 1959), Vol. 3 (Autumn 1958), p. 11. Quoted by Ramsey, *Fabricated Man,* p. 24.

47. Herman J. Muller, "Better Genes for Tomorrow," p. 315, cited by Ramsey, *Fabricated Man,* p. 25.

48. Ramsey, *Fabricated Man,* pp. 19, 26.

49. See McCormick, *How Brave a New World?,* pp. 287f.

50. Ramsey, *Fabricated Man,* p. 89.

51. Karl Barth, *Christ and Adam* (Harper & Row, 1957), p. 29.

52. Gustafson, *Theology and Christian Ethics,* p. 243.

53. Lehmann, *Ethics in a Christian Context,* p. 122.

54. Ibid., p. 123.

55. E. M. B. Greene, *The Meaning of Salvation* (Westminster Press, 1965), pp. 153–189.

56. See Jürgen Moltmann, *The Future of Creation,* trans. Margaret Kohl (London: SCM Press, 1979), p. 45.

57. Ibid., p. 47.

58. Ibid.

59. See Jürgen Moltmann, *The Theology of Hope,* trans. James W. Leitch (Harper & Row, 1962), p. 16.

60. Hick, *Evil and the God of Love,* pp. 207f.

61. Pierre Teilhard de Chardin, *The Future of Man,* trans. Norman Denny (Harper & Row, 1964), pp. 122f.

62. Moltmann, *Theology of Hope,* pp. 222f.

63. Ibid., p. 329.

64. Ibid., p. 18.

65. Wolfhart Pannenberg, *Theology and the Kingdom of God,* ed. Richard John Neuhaus (Westminster Press, 1979), p. 116.

66. Jürgen Moltmann, *The Church in the Power of the Spirit,* trans. Margaret Kohl (Harper & Row, 1977), p. 275.

67. Moltmann, *Theology of Hope,* p. 335.

68. Ibid., p. 337, and Moltmann, *The Church in the Power of the Spirit,* pp. 376f.

69. Ramsey, *Fabricated Man,* p. 29.

70. Moltmann, *Theology of Hope,* p. 22.

71. Ibid., p. 335.

72. Moltmann, *The Church in the Power of the Spirit,* pp. 50f.

73. Pierre Teilhard de Chardin, *The Phenomenon of Man,* trans. Bernard Wall (Harper & Brothers, 1959), pp. 282–283.

74. C. Everett Koop, "Deception on Demand," *Moody Monthly,* Vol. 80 (May 1980), p. 27.

75. See Paul Althaus, *The Ethics of Martin Luther* (Fortress Press, 1972), p. 96, no. 83, who cites *Luther's Works,* 45:396–397.

76. Jürgen Moltmann, *Hope and Planning,* trans. Margaret Clarkson (Harper & Row, 1971), p. 179.

77. Teilhard de Chardin, *Future of Man,* p. 299.

78. Ramsey, *Fabricated Man,* p. 17.

79. Teilhard de Chardin, *The Phenomenon of Man,* pp. 282–283.

80. Fletcher, *The Ethics of Genetic Control,* p. 56.

81. See Schaeffer and Koop, *Whatever Happened to the Human Race?,* p. 86.

82. Reinhold Niebuhr, *The Nature and Destiny of Man,* Vol. 2, p. 166.

83. Moltmann, *Man,* p. 26.

84. Leon R. Kass, "The New Biology: What Price Relieving Man's Estate?" *Science,* Nov. 19, 1971, p. 781.

85. Moltmann, *Man,* p. 26.

86. Lewis, *The Abolition of Man,* p. 35.

87. Moltmann, *Man,* p. 57.

88. Muller, "Genetic Progress by Voluntarily Conducted Germinal Choice," in Jersild and Johnson (eds.), *Moral Issues and Christian Response,* p. 431.

89. Gabriel Fackre, "Ethical Guidelines for the Control of Life," *Christianity and Crisis,* March 31, 1969, cited in Jersild and Johnson (eds.), *Moral Issues and Christian Response,* p. 438.

90. Ibid.

SUBJECT AND NAME INDEX

SCRIPTURE INDEX